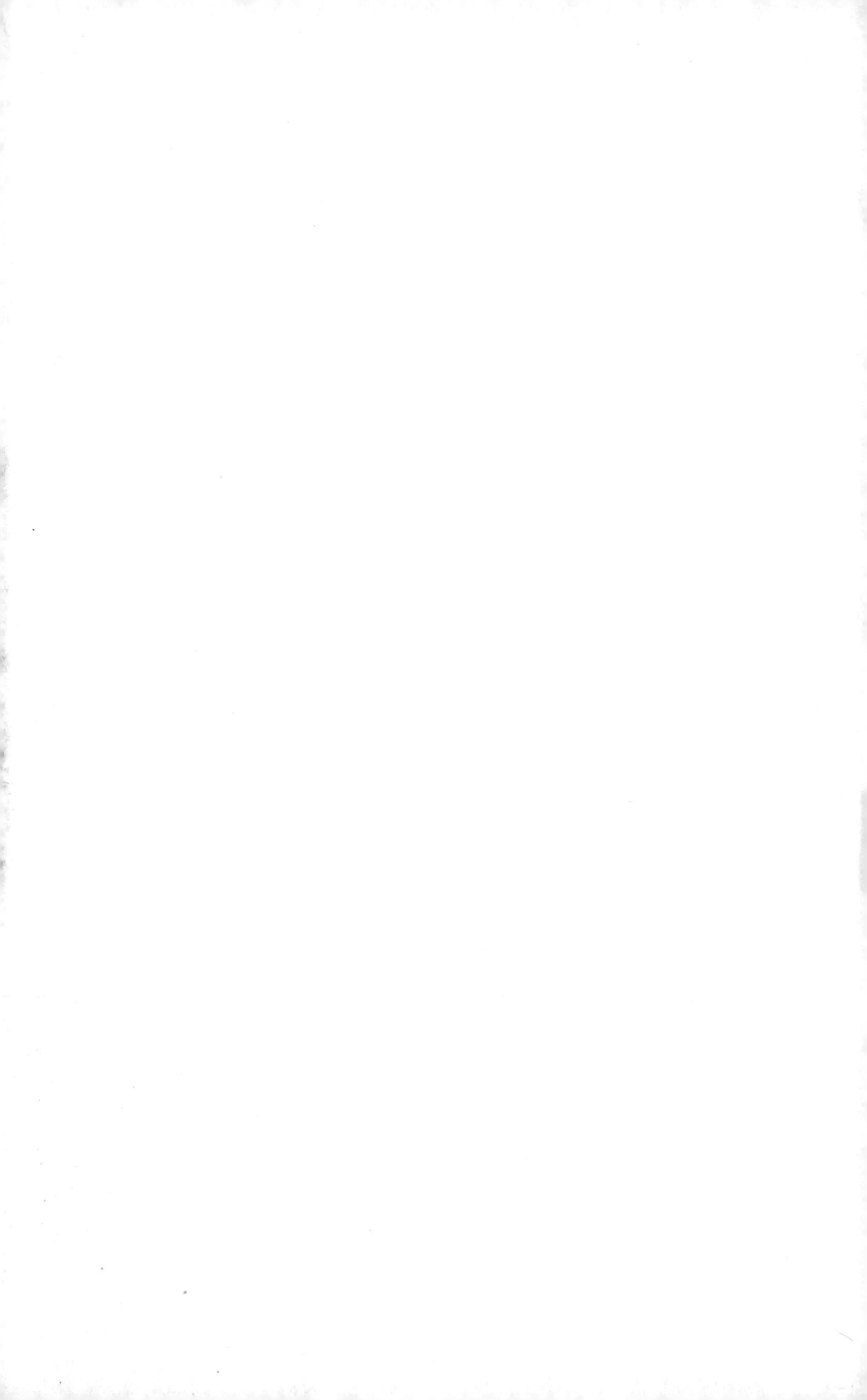

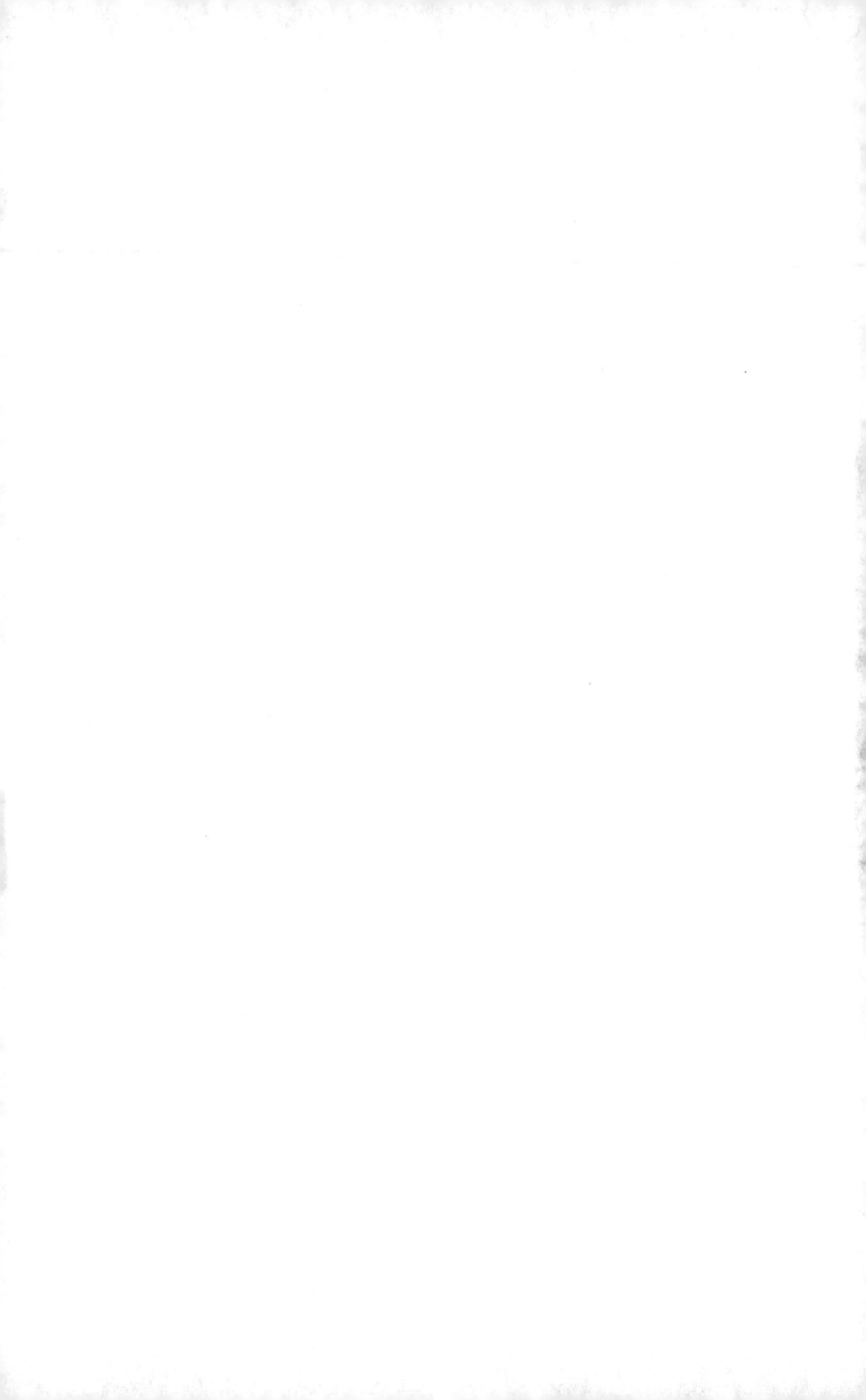

NATURE'S DIET

NATURE'S DIET

Heal Your Body and Stay Healthy by Following Nature's Simple 21 Day Plan

ANDREW IVERSON, N.D.

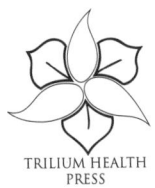

TRILIUM HEALTH
PRESS

Published in the United States of America
by TRILIUM HEALTH PRESS
Tacoma, Washington
www.triliumhealth.com

Printed in the United States of America.

ISBN 978-0-9844724-0-6 (hardcover)

Book design by Matautia Design
www.matautiadesign.com

Special thanks to NATURE'S DIET editors:
Cate Montana and Michael Carroll

Library of Congress Control Number: 2010925620

DISCLAIMER: The material in this book is not a substitute for medical advice or treatment prescribed by your physician. It is provided as a resource for information and education based on the research and experience of Dr. Iverson and the associated community. Dr. Iverson recommends making health decisions based on scientific research by a qualified health care professional. Take nutritional supplements or herbal medicines only at the advice of your physician. The contents are the opinions of Dr. Iverson, unless noted otherwise.

I am in deepest gratitude to my mentor and dear friend, Dr. Kenneth Meadows who first taught me the ways of Nature's Healing Path.

Ken- because of your selflessness and willingness to share your knowledge, your legacy will continue to touch people through these words and beyond. I dedicate this work to you and all the teachers in my life that have contributed their own part to this special book.

"Everything that Man needs for good health and healing is provided in Nature"

Paracelsus, the Father of Pharmacology

CONTENTS

"*Everyone has a doctor in him or her; we just have to help it in its work.*
The natural healing force within each one of us
is the greatest force in getting well.
Our food should be our medicine. Our medicine should be our food."

Hippocrates, The Father of Medicine

Vis Medicatrix Naturae
The Healing Power of Nature

Have you considered the possibility that your body can heal itself?

The first medical doctor, Hippocrates, referred to a *power within the body* that was responsible for healing. This was referred to as the "Healing Power of Nature" or the *Vis Medicatrix Naturae*. As a physician, Hippocrates felt the role of doctors was to assist the natural tendency of the body to heal itself. In that time, doctors like Hippocrates did this by providing the body with the nutrition it needed to regenerate and by removing the obstacles that prevented the body from cure. The doctors of that era believed Nature was both the physician and the healer of the disease. This perspective was the basis of the movement "Nature Cure," a holistic approach based on nutrition and detoxification. How different was this approach taken by our first medical doctors compared to our medical model of today?

Today, billions of dollars are spent in medical research seeking that miracle drug that will cure a specific disease. Science looks to the intricate aspects of a single gene that can be altered or the single chemical that can be synthesized to cure the diseases it studies. Through these efforts, science has become so focused on the minute components of disease, it has lost sight of the original premise upon which Hippocrates founded medicine: *Vis Medicatrix Naturae*. We forget that all around us Nature continues to regenerate and replenish itself. We forget that our body is also a part of this circle of life and it too has the same natural healing capacity; if we provide it what it needs.

In searching to find "the cure", science proves repeatedly what your grandmother's grandmother knew all along: *you can't improve on Nature*. We hear a breaking news flash that science *finally proves* that being active is good for your heart or antioxidants from plants protect against cancer or sunshine is important for strong bones. Science has taken millennia to "prove" basic concepts that have always been true in Nature; concepts which have always been beneficial for the body.

Somehow, somewhere, your great-great-grandmother's common-sense was lost among all this scientific jargon. "Harold, eat your veggies, and drink your water, and get up and move your bottom off the bench, and get some sun, and have fun, and don't sweat the small stuff, and do unto others as you'd have done unto you!" Why don't we follow the sound advice of our forefathers? Our own medical establishment acknowledges Hippocrates as the Father of Medicine but doesn't follow his teachings: Nature Cures.

Even the ancient biblical texts indicate that despite progressive technology and new discoveries nothing is really "new". Everything that is "discovered" has always been here ready to be acknowledged; it just needed someone to desire the knowledge enough to seek the answer.

"There is no new thing under the sun."[1]

"All knowledge is presently with us, all answers are here for us to be enlightened. Just ask and ye shall receive, seek and ye shall find, knock and it shall be opened unto you."[2]

Clearly these words have been around for thousands of years and yet we continue to look for answers to questions that have already been answered for us.

Every answer for our healing is here in front of us if we just pay attention and become aware. Nature beckons us to open our eyes and our ears and observe so that the answers may unfold. Nature is just waiting for the observant few to notice. You do not need to wait any longer for science to prove what Nature is clearly showing you.

This book will guide and teach you how to minimize the main

contributors of disease by following Nature's healing path. It will explain how the causes of illness can be attributed to one or more of the following:

1) Genetic makeup (the card we were dealt)
2) Nutrition and Hydration deficiencies and excesses
3) Chemical toxins and allergic responses
4) Pathogenic causes:
   viruses, bacteria, fungus, yeast, parasites, etc
5) Structural dysfunction affecting joints, muscles, and nerves
6) Electromagnetic interferences
7) Stress and Emotional traumas

Isn't it interesting that these main contributors to disease are highly preventable? By identifying the causes of disease, you have the power to make the changes that will create health. You have the power to build your own wellness by educating yourself on your body's needs. You have the power to become as healthy as you can possibly be. Your doctor can not create health for you; *your primary health care provider is YOU!*

I first decided to write this book because I realized there was a huge need to educate my patients on basic nutrition and wellness. I realized that *so many of my patients would not have needed to come see me at all if they had just simply followed the principles of good eating and healthy living.* Many of us were not taught by our parents what foods to eat in order to be healthy. Teaching our children about good nutrition is a practice that has been lost with our great grandparents. Now though, more than ever, I see a revival of people that want to do the best they can to care for their bodies and their families. I knew that I had to write this book to share what I had learned from my teacher and from my own clinical practice. I knew I had to share what Nature has taught me and pass it onto others so that we won't forget how to live in health and harmony with the planet.

This is a guidebook on how to live according to Nature's principles. It is a book for all of you; readers and non-readers alike. It is a book for both the intellectuals of health and for those who would never have picked up this book if it wasn't recommended to them. It has been written to explain scientific concepts to a large audience from many walks of life in a way that creates intrigue and a thirst for more information. The book will not go into complex scientific details but rather keep the concepts simple and applicable to your daily life.

Are you seeking? Do you want the door do be opened unto you? Let's take a walk down Nature's path. The messages that unfold in the pages of this book are inspired and guided by her wisdom. They are based on the natural scientific laws of physics, chemistry and biology as a whole. They are the application of knowledge received by observing Mother Nature: the plants and animals.

Today, you are invited to take the first step toward a 21 day change for a new life. If it takes 21 days to create a new habit, then let this be its beginning. If you have been having trouble with your weight, feeling fatigued most of the time, or just wanting to give up bad habits and start anew, this is the time to make a change!

Start by simply reading a chapter each day and following the steps for that day. Each day offers something new. These are simple steps that will move you down Nature's intended path to optimal health and harmony.

The first doctor Hippocrates knew that Nature held the answers to our physical, emotional, and spiritual health. These answers have always been here, surrounding us, just waiting for us to discover their subtle truths. All around us wisdom is offered for those willing to be still and observe and listen to Nature's answers to our questions. As Albert Einstein once said,

"Look deep into Nature and understand everything else better."

[1] Ecclesiastes 1:9
[2] Matthew 7:1-8

Introduction
The Student Meets the Teacher

I had it all planned. I would attend the University of Washington and obtain a dual degree in accounting and political science. I would then attend law school, become a lawyer and look to the political arena. I wanted to make my family and friends proud as they were urging me to run for office and become the next representative, senator, or even president of the United States.

There was only one problem. I was miserable. Dreams can crumble easily when one isn't happy in one's own life. I had graduated from high school among the top of my class. However, in my first year of university I found the courses to be more difficult than I had ever imagined and I was not doing well. The classes were not only incredibly demanding but I was also not accustomed to fiercely competitive classmates who seemed willing to cut anyone's throat in order to advance themselves. Most troubling of all, I felt completely uninterested in the subject matter.

These classes were dull, highly analytical, heavy with equations and concepts that were completely foreign to me, and not applicable to my life. I had no idea what I was getting myself into when I first signed up for these classes. I knew nothing about accounting, economics, or political science, but I did know that if I was to have a chance to accomplish what was expected of me, I'd have to do well in these subjects. I was negotiating a very slippery slope and it seemed no matter how hard I dug in with my nails, I just kept sliding. I was the achiever, the first born, the scholar, the ASB president and well-spoken diplomat; a failed student I was not.

When I came home on the weekends my family noticed my stress. They offered what assistance and support they could but the only one who could fight the battle was me. One day my mother offered a rather strange piece of advice. "I think you should get your body chemistry tested. Maybe there are some nutrients that your body is missing so that you can better handle the stress of school. Besides, I really want you to meet this man. He is a special kind of doctor called a *naturopath*. It was such an enlightening appointment and I learned so much about my body that no doctor had ever taught me before. Who knows, let's just see if he can help you too," my mother urged.

∞∞∞∞

My mother had seen improvements in her own health since seeing this "natural doctor" and starting her new "health kick." As a young woman she had been afflicted with adult acne which was painful and made her feel self conscious. She also had a long history of digestive complaints including severe bouts of abdominal pain and constipation. Her energy was low and her lack of drive was affecting her ability to be an active young woman with three energetic children and a husband to care for.

It was a dentist who first suggested her teeth could be the cause of her symptoms. He advised her to remove the dozens of mercury amalgam fillings that were in almost all her teeth. Laboratory testing proved that indeed the fillings were leaching metals into her body, as she tested for very high levels of mercury. Because of these elevated levels, her dentist suggested she see a holistically-minded doctor to detoxify from them. She had never heard of a holistic or natural-minded doctor. Her current family physician was conventionally trained and knew nothing about nutrition or subtle mercury poisoning, much less how to detoxify from it. The doctor's only answer for her was to prescribe more drugs, which she neither wanted nor noticed any benefit from.

So, she sought the assistance of multiple health-oriented practitioners who specialized in treating the whole person, not just the symptoms. She saw chiropractors, massage therapists, craniosacral therapists, acupuncturists, herbalists, nutritionists, and holistic physicians like Chinese doctors and a naturopath. A naturopathic doctor uses the same labs and physical exams as a conventional medical doctor, but instead of initially prescribing drugs to treat the condition, they first prescribe dietary changes and natural medicines. These health-oriented practitioners focused on improving my mother's health through diet and nutrition, lifestyle changes, botanical herbal medicine, homeopathy, hydrotherapy, psychological counseling, exercise, and stretching protocols.

I remember those early years as she experimented on not just herself but the whole family as she prepared for us these strange "organic health" foods. They tasted fibrous and bland and weren't too pretty to look at either. Our home would be filled with the strange smells of mushrooms, roots, leaves, bark and unfamiliar berries as she boiled her Chinese herbal teas every night. We thought she had definitely lost her mind as she would dispense pills from the dozens of bottles of supplements that she took faithfully at each meal.

She wasn't particularly excited about all these new food changes either. She was a "sweet-aholic" and giving up her "treats" along with her weekly gallon of cow's milk was not a welcome thought. (Did I mention she grew up on a dairy farm? Some habits die hard.) She persevered because interestingly enough she saw positive changes. For the first time in her adult life her symptoms were actually improving. Her energy was coming back and her stomach no longer ached and cramped after meals. Her digestion was the best in her life with more regular bowel movements. Even her acne was clearing. Her hard work was paying off and she became the living example of healing through natural methods. Today, my mother has none of these original symptoms. She has her health back and looks years younger than her biological age.

Through her example, I decided to take my mother's advice and made an appointment to see this old doc. And this is where my journey began…

ooooo

It was an odd setting for a "doctor" alright. This so called "clinic" was not what I was typically used to as a medical clinic; it was someone's house!

"Oh God," I said to myself, "my mother has really lost it. She can't be serious? This has to be a joke. She's been led to believe that a doctor would work in a place like this?"

I slowly opened the door, not knowing whether to knock or not, and poked my head through the crack, "Hello? Dr. Meadows?"

It was a long pause. I must have had the wrong place. Someone is certainly going to call the cops on me for breaking into his home.

"Hello? ... Dr. Meadows?" I called out, my voice cracking from nervousness.

"Yes, come in please," I heard an older man's voice. He entered from the back room and stood there smiling softly at me. He was a silver haired gentleman wearing a classic 70's style tan suit and looking out from rounded wire spectacles. He kindly reached out his warm hands and took mine into his, "I've heard so much about you, grand man. My name is Ken."

It was an instant feeling of kinship. He seemed so familiar to me I felt as if I had always known him. Still shaking his hand and smiling he asked me to please sit down.

He began by sharing about himself. He had come from Akron, Ohio and worked for many years as a chemist for Goodyear Tire Company. He went on to say how he had been led to natural medicine in the 1960's after hearing lectures, reading books, and attending retreats given by original health pioneers Dr. Paavo Airola, Dr. John Christopher, Dr. Bernard Jensen, and Dr. Norman Walker, among others. He witnessed miraculous healings in the patients who followed their nutritional guidelines. He also saw positive changes in his own body and that inspired him to emulate his mentors and become a healer himself. He followed his heart and left Goodyear to acquire additional training in biochemistry and a degree in Naturopathy.

Along the way he encountered a biochemist mathematician by the name of Carey Reams. He went on to study for eight years with Dr. Reams at his health retreats in Virginia. He explained how Dr. Reams had used a mathematical equation to determine the energetic needs of the body, an equation which was related to Einstein's famous equation $E=mc^2$. The "m" stood for "mass" which is represented as "food" and which is broken down into "E" or "energy." "You live off the energy of the food, not just from the food itself. All food has to be converted into energy for you to utilize it," he said. He was going to determine how my body was turning food into energy by analyzing my urine and saliva samples.

ooooo

He rocked in his chair as he told me how the body is composed of the same substances as the Earth. "We are made of oxygen, hydrogen, carbon, nitrogen, sulfur, and dozens and dozens of elements and minerals. If we are deficient in even one of these elements, we lose energy. A loss of energy means less fuel for the body's repair mechanisms and this can result in illness and disease," he said with great knowingness.

"In addition to losing energy from nutritional deficiencies, the body can also lose energy by toxins overloading the system. These toxins can come from the chemicals in our environment or even drugs that people use as medicine. They can also come from the chemicals that are added to our food to make them taste better or last longer. A healthy body also produces toxins on a daily basis as waste products. If we lose our ability to eliminate these toxins, we will also lose energy."

When he wanted me to really understand an important point he would raise his voice and speak with annunciation, *"Our overall health and vitality is highly determined by the ability to take in and assimilate nutrition and the ability to excrete and eliminate wastes and toxins."*

He continued to rock back and forth and talk for a long time, but I was in no way bored. What he was teaching made inherent sense to me and I was completely fascinated. He went on to say that our physical health can also be affected by non-material influences like our mental attitude. He taught that we can create health by using our minds to focus on the positive or we can create illness with "mental toxicity" by basking in thoughts of negativity and stress.

"Your perception of stress in your life as well as your feelings and emotions contribute to your mental state. Too much 'dis'-'ease' can eventually create in the body real life DISEASE. This is the root cause of much illness," he taught, "not being at 'ease' with life." I felt like he was reading my soul. He was saying exactly what I needed to hear at that exact moment in my life.

He continued, "Persistent feelings of worthlessness, guilt, fear, anger, rejection, hopelessness, helplessness, and a sense of being overwhelmed by life can eventually show up as physical symptoms in the body. I have seen these emotions lead to anxiety, depression, insomnia, headaches, stomach aches, skin conditions, and body aches to name a few," he said.

"You have to consider not just the food you put in your mouth but the thoughts you feed your mind. Your mind is listening to your every word! Your mind hears your every thought!" he would say fervently. "If you think and speak negatively or think poorly of yourself, your brain will respond to that by giving you more of the same. In other words, you won't be able to get ahead and crawl out of your misery. *You are what you think!*"

Wow! I hung on every word. I couldn't get enough. It was completely fascinating to me and made complete sense when I related it to my former studies on psychology and physiology...and, "coincidentally" it was as if he knew what I was going through at school. It was as if he was telling me exactly what it was I needed to do to heal that "dis"-"eased" part of my life.

ooooo

He took samples of my urine and saliva and he proceeded to interpret the results of the tests. They showed that my digestion was slow and inefficient at breaking down proteins into amino acids. It also showed I was not assimilating my minerals and vitamins as I should because I was not combusting my food into energy efficiently. Insufficient nutrition from my food could be the explanation for my low energy level and my anxiety in stressful situations.

He had me stick out my tongue while he did a Chinese tongue reading. He noted where there were cracks, colors, and coatings that indicated organ stress. Then he looked into my eyes to read the reflexes in the iris and the sclera which correlated with organs in the body which could be losing energy. Finally he looked at the markings on my fingernails and noted the shape of my face and the stature of my body, techniques used in both Chinese medicine and Ayurvedic medicine from India.

In a few minutes Ken had written a list of organ reflexes and physical health tendencies based on what he found by reading my eyes, tongue and body shape. He combined these findings with the results from the labs and he designed a treatment protocol. He selected specific foods, various minerals and nutrients, and chose botanical medicine in the form of herbal teas to create a program specifically for my unique body chemistry.

It was all so intriguing and it made so much sense. As a little boy I wanted to be a doctor but I never knew that there was a doctor that treated in this way - using the medicine that Nature provided us. This visit with Ken had given me new inspiration about medicine. The hours we spent together flew by as I was thirsting for more and more. "If you want me to teach you more come back tomorrow at 3 pm." It was a deal. I went home excited to share what I had learned and even more eager to see what tomorrow would hold.

ooooo

It became a ritual, our weekend meetings; I would sit and take notes while Ken talked at length while rocking back and forth in his chair. I would stay late into the night and was completely fascinated by the accounts of healing miracles he had witnessed at the health retreats lead by Dr. Carey Reams. People came there as a last resort, having turned away from conventional medicine, which had led them to believe nothing could be done for them. I learned that many of them recovered by following the simple healing practices of good nutrition, botanical medicine, and hydrotherapy.

Ken would fondly share the teachings of a mentor teacher under whom he studied for twelve years and who had greatly inspired his calling to natural medicine. This teacher was a Shaolin monk named Master Ong who taught him how to harness the life force energy found within all things called "Chi.". He used ancient exercises like Kung Fu and Tai Chi to channel this energy for healing the body.

I would listen in awe as Ken recalled how Master Ong magically appeared in a room without anyone witnessing his entering through the door. He chuckled as he told how Master Ong would jump from a table onto an egg without cracking its shell. He accounted with amazement how the Master could harness Chi energy and launch students across the room without ever touching them physically. Master Ong was a Kung Fu Master, he was not a fairy tale story. Ken wanted me to understand that the very same energy Master Ong utilized to perform these miracles could be channeled by any person to create healing miracles in his or her body.

He sent me back to university with a half dozen different books each week. Their subjects ranged from nutrition, biochemistry, anatomy, herbal medicine, massage, acupuncture, homeopathy, cleansing, and fasting, to psychology, sociology, counseling, placebos, mind-over-matter, world religions, death and dying, and spirituality.

"You have to know yourself before you can know others and you have to know God before you can know yourself. It is just as important for you to learn about the mental and the spiritual needs of the person as it is for you to learn about the biochemical and physical needs of the person. You are not just a physical body. You are also a thinking mental body and a feeling spiritual body." Ken had made it very clear to me that a scientist does not leave God out of the equation because science and God are inextricable. They cannot be separated.

∞∞∞∞

I was so excited about what I was learning that I spent more time reading my new books than I spent reading my university assignments. My time was occupied by education of a different sort and it was fun, exciting, and inspiring. My new "class" was filled with subjects which had interested me since my youth. As a boy I couldn't get enough of Nature. I spent almost all my free time in the great outdoors fishing, hunting, raising orphaned baby animals and growing dozens of seedlings of different plant species in my greenhouse.

I would conduct my own "scientific" experiments on frogs' eggs and tadpoles and my pet goldfish. I would cross-pollinate plants to create flowers with new characteristics and cross-breed rabbits to create babies with new colors. Like most young boys I was also completely fascinated by magic and ghost stories. In elementary school I checked out every book in the library which dealt with powers of the mind like ESP, hypnosis, levitation, and moving objects through telekinesis. It seemed that these early childhood fascinations were being re-sparked by my "self-taught" elective course.

∞∞∞∞

Summer came and so did a proposal from my teacher Ken, "Andy, I must pass on my knowledge to someone before I leave this planet. I am proposing that you be my protégé. Would you like for me to teach you the ways of natural medicine?" He asked with great earnestness. I didn't hesitate for a moment. "YES!" The thought of it excited me more than any possibility I had ever known. This was the answer I had been seeking for my future.

So it was that every day I would ride my bicycle to Ken's home-office where I would sit with him and observe him with his patients. I was the fly on the wall and I learned as "Doc Ken," as he was affectionately referred to by his patients, lectured on health and nutrition and biochemistry. I listened as he counseled and I was struck by his gift for expressing compassion for those in states of emotional pain. The words he spoke to his patients were like a soothing elixir. They came from a place deep inside him and were perfectly selected to bring peace, contentment, and healing to the soul of their receiver.

In the beginning, I just sat there in the back of the room, observing and taking notes. Later, Ken taught me to do the laboratory testing to determine the biochemical patterns. After several months he allowed me to write the patient's dietary and supplement recommendations on their prescription sheets. I was catching on fast and it came naturally and easily to me.

That next autumn I returned to school to make the biggest decision of my life. Following my heart, I changed my major from accounting and politics to pre-medicine with a major in neuropsychology (how the brain perceives the world and makes the body work). School became a breeze after that. It was hard for me to believe that I was in the same level of university classes. Now, instead of struggling not to fail, I was getting the top grades in the class with very little memorization effort. I was building upon the knowledge and practical situations I had learned in the clinic with Doc Ken. Interestingly enough, even some professors asked for my opinion on certain subjects from a natural medicine perspective.

I continued to assist Ken on weekends throughout my undergraduate years at the University of Washington. We would usually settle down on the back porch after work and spend the rest of the evening discussing the cases of the day.

I fondly remember staying up late into the night sharing and laughing and ending the evening with a meditation and prayer. Some nights I would stay the night so we could wake before dawn and hike into the dew-filled forest to pray and meditate some more.

Ken's famous words still echo in my ears today, *"Get the guilt out of your life, man!" "You are worthy! You are worth it!"* He taught me the importance of being faithful to my word. He impressed on me the importance of following through on the things you say you'll do. *Be true to the commitments you make to others. Have intention and purpose in your life. Your thoughts are powerful, use them wisely,*" were just a few of his frequently spoken pieces of advice. My teacher was a wise man. He imparted these great truths to me and above all, he lived these by example. Not once did I hear a negative word cross his lips about anybody. He was faithful to his word and he gave every human the benefit of the doubt.

One of these infamous nights Ken said something I'll never forget, "There comes a time when the student shall surpass the teacher. It must be this way for us to evolve as Humanity. The time has come for me to pass the torch to you."

ooooo

And so it was. From that day forward Doc Ken sat in the back of the room as he observed the student he molded from the beginning. Now he observed as I took his place and counseled the patients based on their individual chemistry and physical exam findings. He sat back and felt the emotions that filled the room as I prepared the same space he prepared for his patients. And my patients felt the same comfort and peace to release these emotions as his patients had once released with him.

Every day during the summer and on weekends during the school year, I would see patients with Ken. This went on for all four years, and by the time I entered naturopathic medical school, I had the clinical experience of some of my professors. They often asked me how I had learned to treat a specific condition. It came so naturally to me and I had learned so much from the greatest teacher in life: real life experience! Ken had given me an invaluable gift; the wisdom he imparted to me was the greatest education anyone could have ever asked for.

Today, Ken is no longer with us. He passed the torch so his legacy could live through me. Now, I want to share it with you. This book is a compilation of what I learned from my teacher Ken as well as what I have experienced first-hand in my own clinic. This first book focuses on healing the physical body through nourishment and detoxification. Much of the information here is backed by scientific research although some of it is based on personal clinical experience, observation, and intuition.

It is with great pleasure that I invite you to take a walk with me down a path I discovered for the first time many years ago. My wise old teacher once taught me, *"If you unlock the secrets of Nature... all your answers will be found."* Let's take this walk down "Nature's path" and through the wisdom of a naturopath, Doc Ken, and my own personal clinical experiences, we will unlock Nature's secrets.

Day 1
AWARENESS AWAKENS
The food which crosses my lips

In my own experience, I found I was always more motivated to begin a new project if it was fun and interesting and not too complicated. So with that in mind, let's start this first day simply. There is no need for you to feel overwhelmed. This entire book is going to be a fun and insightful experience.

Your first step today is to practice being aware. Becoming aware of how you are in the world is the first step to understanding yourself and changing your life. If you are unaware of your habits, you are not capable of changing them. If you don't know what you are doing wrong how can you hope to fix it?

You may be surprised to find out that if you asked someone what they had for lunch yesterday they may not be able to remember. You may not remember everything that you put in your mouth today even! Most of us are on some kind of "auto-pilot". We go about our day in a hypnotic fashion, often just going through the motions. Whether we are responding to the mundane tasks at work, driving on the freeway, or even feeding our faces, we tend to "check out" until something of interest sparks our attention and brings us back to the present.

We may not even realize we are snacking and nibbling all day. We eat while busy at work or while we watch television or when we talk on the phone. Little did you know that your lack of present awareness helped you to support the Frito Lay Company as the famous Doritos™ commercial indicates "Bet ya can't eat just one." Largely unconscious and unaware, you eat and eat, not even realizing the whole bag is gone or the whole pizza eaten or the whole gallon of ice cream slurped down.

Why is it that we check out? How can being unaware or going "unconscious" affect your life? Those questions we will address in books to come. Now, we primarily want to understand how to become aware of our food choices so that we can have a positive impact on our health and our waistlines.

Time to Take Notes

So here is the first step in bringing food awareness into your life. *Simply begin by writing down every single thing you put in your mouth and include the amounts of each item you are eating.* This will be the beginning of your diet diary. It may sound overly simple or seem like a waste of time but it serves important purposes. First, it will put your focus back onto the food you consume. This will help you identify the types of foods you are eating and how much of them. This practice becomes increasingly important as you learn more about how different foods affect your health. The best part about writing down your foods is that studies have proven that people who simply write down what they are eating double their weight loss![1] Wow! How is that for a motivator?

It is quite amazing how you can affect your body by simply being aware of your food choices. Bringing in this awareness will help you realize that you are responsible for your health and you are in a powerful position to promote your personal healing. You may even say, as so many others have who started this program, "Wow, I didn't even realize I ate so much junk!" or "I didn't realize that I drink six cups of coffee a day!" This is the first step to bring more awareness into your daily food practice.

How Bad Could it Get?

I don't want you to end up the same way so many of my well-intentioned patients have. They start their new lifestyle program eager and excited to change their life and become healthy, but like most things new and exciting, it eventually fizzles out. In order for this to really work for you as a lasting practice beyond these 21 days, you have to decide to make a COMMITMENT to YOU. You have to make an AGREEMENT with YOU to truly achieve what you want out of your life.

You probably hear this often; someone says, "Yes, I am going to go on a diet. I am going to lose weight. I am going to start exercising and eating right. I am going to get in shape and feel better." The problem is they may say they don't want to be fat, but in reality they have NO PLAN to make these changes happen. They don't have a specific plan outlining how they will achieve their goal. In order to be successful, they have to be specific about their outcome such as, "In order to lose this amount of weight, I must eat this and that, and I will dedicate myself to exercise this many hours and this many days a week."

In addition to a plan, you must also have the motivation or reasoning to follow through with it. If you are someone who fails to lose weight over and over, it is because you may not yet have given yourself a big enough reason to make a change. "So what if I am a little chubby? So what if I am a little more tired? So what if I'm not as sexy or as good looking as I used to be? So what? Nobody is as they get older anyway… right?" The problem with these folks is they have no real motivator. Even though they are overweight and fatigued they are still considered to be "healthy" according to American standards and their doctor. They've never had cancer or diabetes or some other life threatening illness so they have no real "reason" or major motivation to stop living the way they are.

My teacher once said that he was not able to convince anyone of anything if he did not have their trust and their faith. If they trusted him and believed that he could help them, then he had the leverage he needed to help them. He used that leverage to get them motivated to make the changes they needed so they could help themselves.

Often he used the strong belief the patients had in him to pose to them thought provoking questions, such as "What will eventually happen if you don't make these health changes?" "How much worse could your symptoms get if you don't change your life?" "What sicknesses may come to you if you don't take care of your health right now?" "What will you look like in 10 years if you continue this path of destruction?"

What I witnessed is that those patients who actually sat down and took the time to answer these questions honestly were the patients who made EXTREME CHANGES and received EXTREME RESULTS. These were the folks who actually took the time to write down in detail and create a mental picture of *how bad it could really get!* The others who thought about it and let it just fade away into the memories of thoughts didn't have the motivation to keep on their programs. As with any fad, these individuals were on our program for a week and then fell of it like they fell off all the others before ours. As quickly as they came to see us, they left to seek the next magic guru with the next magic pill.

"So how bad could it get if I don't change?" You might ask yourself. Well here is a nice example:

"If I don't make these changes then:"

"If I don't change, my joints will get worse and I will become crippled and could become so handicapped that I lose my freedom to come and go as I please. I will have to depend on other people to help me and that means I will become a burden to others."

"If I don't change, I can see myself becoming prematurely old and my skin will become discolored and wrinkly. I can see my hair turning grey early and even falling out in clumps, making me totally bald."

"If I don't change, my teeth will rot and fall out of my mouth and I will talk like an idiot and look like an old geezer and I'll never be able to eat corn on the cob or apples again."

"If I don't change, I will be fatter than I am now and because I am so overweight I will become depressed. If I am depressed then I won't care and I won't take care of my hygiene and I will smell sour and rotten."

"If I don't change and I become fat and ugly and toothless and smelly, then I will turn away from socializing and become withdrawn and bitter and lose friends and family and all connections with the joy in my life."

How does that sound? What a list of miserable consequences in a miserable existence, and all the result of NOT making the choice to CHANGE today! One of the greatest motivational speakers in the world, Tony Robbins, uses these same techniques to create massive changes in peoples' lives. He teaches that the only way to make lasting lifestyle changes is to make the PAIN of your bad habits greater than the PLEASURE of the foods or the alcohol or smokes or any other vices that imprison you.

If you want to achieve the results you have to dig deep and be so sick and tired of being sick and tired that you scream out like Tony Robbins himself, "That's it! No more! I am not going to take it anymore!" If you don't, then you can join the masses and it will be a guaranteed failure over and over and over again.

This reminds me of a story of one of my patients who told me about a day in which she made a life-changing choice. Leslie was 25 years old and lovely in physical shape and beauty. No one would have ever guessed that a couple years prior she looked like a completely different person. This is what she told me.

"Dr. Iverson, have you ever faced adversity in your life?"

"Well," I responded, "neither myself nor my immediate family has had any life-threatening illnesses or deaths. So I will say no."

"Well, would you believe that a couple years ago I weighed 100 pounds more than I do today?"

I looked at her wide-eyed, "Please tell me how you did it!"

"Actually, one day, simply enough, I just chose not to be fat anymore. I decided that was it. I woke up that morning and said, "From today onwards I will never be fat again. I'm done with it." I told myself that I have lived the experience of what it is like to be obese and I now I am ready to know what it is like to be thin. I no longer needed that experience in that body any longer. I had lived every part of that experience and I owned it. All I did was consciously make the decision to be thin. I have never gone back and I never will."

Leslie became so personally aware of what it felt like to be overweight and became so aware of the PAIN it was causing her that she decided to take extreme steps to change it.

When we make up our minds and choose the path we want to take, there is very little that can stop us. Whether it is trying to break an addiction from food, from substances, or from anything else, we will only be able to do so when we get leverage. Leverage finally comes when we have truly decided that the experience has been fulfilled and we are ready to move onwards to new ones. What are you currently aware of that needs to be changed in your life?

Become Accountable to Others

Studies have also shown that we are much more likely to be accountable to our new lifestyle if we share these health commitments with people close to us in our lives. People are much more likely to follow through with a plan if they write it on paper, sign their names to the bottom and give copies to those whom they respect most. This means that no longer are we out to do this just for ourselves, we are doing it for those people that love and care for us too.

For example, your letter may look something like this:

Dear Mom, I am writing this to tell you that, as your son, I am making major changes to benefit my health as of this date (_____). I am making a commitment to myself and my family so that I may live a healthy happy life. I am dedicating myself to:

1) Following these dietary changes: (list)
2) Following these exercise changes: (list)
3) Eliminating these unhealthy habits: (list)
4) My goal is to lose this much weight by this date: (for example)

Go one step further and share your letter of health commitment and your diet diary with a health-oriented practitioner or personal trainer so they can give you even more feedback. It allows the practitioner to see what foods in your diet could be contributing to weight gain, potential allergic responses, and poor health. Having this "coach" read your diary means you are more accountable for what you are eating.

Naturally, we want to look good in the eyes of others, so if we are sharing our diet diary with someone else, we will more than likely want to eat foods we know our coaches would approve of. Having such a coach and having our friends and family to support us and keep us motivated can help bring greater results than we've ever seen before.

Try it out! It is simple, effective and CHEAP! Who could ask for a better alternative to a weight loss program in economic times like this, right? Now just go do it! Don't just read about doing it... to really be effective, you have to actively participate and just do it! (Thanks, Nike!) Okay... start now and we will resume tomorrow.

[1]Time, 2008 Aug 4, Gupta PMID 18831096 =Victor J. Stevens, Ph.D., senior investigator, Kaiser Permanente Center for Healthy Research, Portland, Ore.; Keith Bachman, M.D., weight management specialist, Kaiser Permanente Care Management Institute, Portland, Ore.; American Journal of Preventive Medicine Volume 35, Issue 2, Pages 118-126 (August 2008)

START TODAY:

- To start the practice of awareness and to be effective in doing it; please write down everything that goes in your mouth and the amount that was consumed. This will need to be done diligently for the entire 21 days.

- Secondly, take the time to write down in detail what could happen in the future if you don't make extreme changes now. Write down every single detail from your physical health to your mental well being. Create the ugliest, scariest picture of how you could end up if you don't change now. (Think of it as Scrooge seeing his future in 'A Christmas Carol' and dramatically changing his life afterwards!)

- Finally, write letters to your loved ones declaring what health changes you are making and the commitment you are making to yourself and to them. Be accountable! Share your letter and your diary with a health-minded practitioner so he or she can be your support coach along the way.

Summary: This is what I'm doing up to this point, each day adds onto the next

Day 1: AWARENESS AWAKENS: keep a diary of my foods, detailed description of what could happen if I don't change, write a letter of my commitment and accountability.

Day 2
Water – the Liquid of Life

You are off to a great start by writing down the foods you are eating. Are you becoming more aware of your food choices and amounts? Did you take the time to write how about how bad it could get if you don't change right now? Did you write your commitment letter to your loved ones? If you haven't done it, get to it... this is just as important as anything else I'm about to teach. Without making a true commitment then you are only "wanting" to get well instead of "actively pursuing" wellness. As Mick Jagger reminds us so well, "You can't always get what you want."

On your second day, we will add one more healthy habit. I have found in my clinic that my patients would be more likely to create lasting health changes if I didn't slash and burn all their unhealthy habits right away. In fact, I found that instead of taking away their vices, I had better luck with their making lasting changes by instead *adding in* several good ones first. Eventually by adding in more and more and more good choices, there is hardly any room for the not-so-good habits because they have been crowded out by the healthy habits.

Today, the focus is to become conscious about liquids. Water is Nature's universal solvent, which means it has the ability to mix with substances to create a solution. It can mix with your food to bring minerals, vitamins and other nutrients into your cells. Likewise, it can also mix with your body's waste products such as acids, urea, and toxins to carry them out. Therefore water is essential to bring nutrition into your cells and carry the waste out of your body's cells.

Little does one stop to wonder how important water really is to the body. Consider that your body is made up of approximately 60% water. Isn't it an interesting coincidence that is about the same proportion of water that is covering the EARTH? We may be more like "our Mother" than we thought. Think of what is left of the human body after one is cremated, a small box of ashes which are mostly minerals. We'll talk about the essentials of minerals later. Because water composes such a large percentage of the body, it would be expected that if we were without water, we may have some serious issues.

Water is essential for brain functions, such as maintaining a sharp memory and quick wit because the brain itself is about 75% water and it depends on an ample supply for complex functioning and thinking quickly on its feet. In fact, not just the brain but the heart, the lungs, the liver, the kidneys and all the muscles are soaking in 75% to 85% water! This means that the most vital organs running the most vital processes are first and foremost dependent on the solvent of Nature to make sure they are functioning properly. Water is the main component of any fluid in your body. Water is essential for creating the lubrication in joints that give us smooth and comfortable movement. It is what makes up the digestive juices in your gut so you can break down food and maintain a healthy weight. It is the main component of your saliva so you can have sweet breath and beautiful teeth. It is the major part of sweat, helping to clean the impurities from your skin and giving you a glowing and youthful complexion. The tears which lubricate your eyes are made from water to keep them from getting too dry. It is the main component in your blood, helping it carry oxygen so you have great energy and excellent circulation. Circulation is vital for everything from healthy memory to a healthy heart and, of course, a healthy sex life! Any of these areas mentioned need improvement in you??

Interestingly, most of my patients are not getting enough water to drink but are getting more than enough food to eat. They seem to be having persistent cravings for food or treats throughout the day.

As humans, we commonly mistake our need for drinking more water as a craving for food. Instead of putting in pure water, a cleansing liquid free of calories, we continue to snack and nibble until we are satisfied. Just sipping on water throughout the day fulfills the body's need and can help many people curb these food cravings.

As a clinician, I've been impressed by the miraculous results I've seen simply when a body consumes regular amounts of purified water. I feel this is due to the positive effect water has on lessening inflammation in the body. Science is proposing that the start of all disease is due to inflammation of the cells. Well, think of what inflammation is: it's hot and red and burning. Think of inflammation as though the body is on FIRE! And, how do you put out a fire? Yes! Water! The answers are always there; all we have to do is look to Nature and see how It puts out fiery inflammation. Is it no wonder my patients see their joint pains lessening, their hot-acid fire bellies cooling down, their constipation improving, their skin softening and clearing, their persistent urinary and candida infections disappearing and their energy increasing?

Water is Like No Other Liquid on Earth

Water is a special liquid. No other liquid can compare to it. Even though fruit juices, sport drinks such as Gatorade™ and Powerade™, energy drinks such as Red Bull™ and Rock Star™, soft drinks, tea, coffee and alcohol all have water in them, they are not natural or healthful sources of getting your water. These drinks can act as diuretics, which actually dehydrate your body causing it to lose more water than it is consuming. Of course, several of them are also high in sugar and tainted with artificial chemicals such as dyes and flavorings, not to mention loaded with nervous system stimulants such as caffeine which can create other health problems.

These fluids also create extra work for your body. It takes energy for the body to separate the water from the rest of the ingredients in these liquids. It must do this before it can use the remaining water for cellular functions. This extra step of filtering the fluids is not an efficient use of energy. Remember: Nature follows the Laws of Physics and takes the *path of least resistance*.[1] This means it would prefer to conserve energy and take the route which is the least amount of work. Don't make your body work so hard for something so simple! Give it pure water!

Yes it is hard to believe but even fruit juice is not a healthy choice! Juice is not a natural food! You will not find it in Nature! You cannot find a tree dispensing fruit juice ready to drink can you? Juice is actually processed liquid which has been separated from its natural fibers and contains very concentrated amounts of sugar. It can be as damaging as drinking soda because of its high sugar content. This, too, is a problem for vegetable juices like carrot juice, which many health food junkies think is a health food. We'll talk more about this later on the subject of fruit.

Nature has provided us with all the clues we need to understand the proper fluid intake for our bodies. All we have to do is open our awareness and look to what Nature is doing. Although Willy Wonka may have had fountains flowing with grape juice or rivers of root beer... as far as currently known...there are no such things found in Nature. Water is the common link that all living beings share together.

Wild animals drink 100% water 100% of the time, unless they are babies drinking breast milk or my buddy's puppy who has found a taste for beer! The amount each animal drinks is different depending upon the species and the climate in which it lives. An animal's need for water isn't as high as their human counterparts, but then, they also aren't eating at Taco Bell, Pizza Hut, McDonald's, or Ben & Jerry's on a regular basis either. They consume no foods containing salt, seasonings, MSG or sauces. Animals do not drink dehydrating fluids like alcohol, coffee, or soda and they eat foods that have a higher content of natural water such as plants and raw flesh. Their need to flush out the toxic by-products of artificial flavoring and coloring is not necessary because they do not consume them.

Nature's Purification of Water

Wild animals drink water provided by Nature in the form of rain or from a spring or glacier river source. Nature's water supply goes through a natural purification process by one of several methods. Rain water is actually distilled water, purified from the evaporated water which accumulates as clouds. Spring water is naturally filtered as it percolates through the sediment in the earth. Glacier water is melted snow water that cuts through the mountainside, creating milk-water that is loaded with micro-sized trace minerals that it carries into the valley as rivers.

Nature even cleans its water of the electromagnetic memories of whatever was in contact with it before we drink it. Electromagnetic "memory" refers to the frequency or vibrational energy of the water. Every plant and animal and rock has a specific vibrational frequency or energy unique to itself. Even poisons and toxins carry their own vibrational frequency. Water is a unique liquid that has an ability to hold the frequency, or "remember" whatever it was previously in contact with . This frequency is stored in water as a memory called resonance[2]. Water which is filtered may be free of the chemical contaminants, but it still has the resonant "memory" or resonant frequency of whatever was in it before it was filtered. Your water could have the memory of pesticides, heavy metals, medications, industrial solvents, human waste, and the memory of any other creature that drank it and urinated it out prior to your drinking it!

What? Does that sound disgusting to drink recycled water? Yes, it sounds much worse than ABC gum. (Already Been Chewed, for those that remember back to second grade). But, remember that all the water that is on the planet right now, is the very same water that has always been here during the history of the earth. It is not re-created or destroyed, it just changes its form and is recycled beneath this greenhouse bubble around the earth which we call the atmosphere. The same water you are drinking today is the same water the dinosaurs and cave men and wooly mammoths once drank! Nature has created a perfect system for recycling its water supply by filtering it through rain distillation or spring percolation to remove the chemical contaminants and it has even devised a way to remove these former memories.

Think of the river currents creating millions of spinning vortices as the water moves rapidly down river beds. These little vortices spin so quickly that they produce an electromagnetic charge across the vortex funnel. This charge electrically clears the water of the memory of any substance or anything that was in contact with the water prior. This gives you pristine and electrically neutral water which no longer has the memory of Tyrannosaurus Rex or your ancestors like Fred Flintstone.

The City's Idea of Water Purification

The water you choose for you and your family should mimic Nature as closely as possible. It should be from a clean source; this means that tap water, unless it is from a well, is not recommended. City water is treated with chlorine and fluoride both of which are well-known to be oxidizing agents (which mean they accelerate aging.) An example of oxidation is what happens when metallic iron is exposed to the air: yes, it rusts! When chlorine is added to our water, it combines with other chemicals to form compounds with long names like disinfection by-products (DBPs), trihalomethanes (THMs), haloacetic acids (HAA), trichloroethylene (TCE) and chloroform, all of which are known carcinogens. These chlorine by-products accelerate the production of free radicals in your body causing cell damage and have been implicated in heart disease and even some types of cancers.

The most harmful exposure to chlorine is due to the inhalation of steam and skin absorption while showering. The heat from a shower causes even more absorption of the chlorine and other chemicals because it opens the pores in your skin. Some sources say the steam inhaled while showering can contain 10-50 times more harmful chemicals than drinking the same tap water. This is because chlorine and most other contaminants vaporize much faster at a higher temperature. Chemicals become more dangerous when inhaled than when swallowed because upon inhalation they pass directly into your bloodstream, bypassing the detoxifying function of the liver. Chlorine vapors are known to be a strong irritant to the sensitive bronchial passages in our lungs and can exacerbate the respiratory conditions asthma and bronchitis.

Fluoride is a subject of great debate particularly because conventional medical dogma considers it a key element for dental health. Fluoride is actually as toxic as the heavy metal lead to humans although the naturally occurring form of calcium fluoride is relatively harmless because it is not easily assimilated and Nature supplies it in minute quantities. Sodium fluoride is an industrial waste product which is added to water and used in dental treatments to prevent tooth decay. One way it does this is by poisoning the bacteria in your mouth through enzyme inhibition. The bad news is that it poisons the cells in your body as well. It is a powerful central nervous system toxin and can affect brain function even in small quantities. Studies show that fluoride is associated with reduced cognitive and learning abilities in children.[3]

The purpose of adding fluoride to our drinking water was to harden teeth and thus prevent cavities. Now it is known that too much of a supposed good thing can cause dental and skeletal fluorosis. In this condition, the teeth and bone become porous with little holes. These little holes weaken the tooth's enamel resulting in deformities. It causes the bones to become brittle and makes them susceptible to fracture as well as increases the risk of bone cancer or osteosarcoma. Large studies conducted by the National Institute of Dental Research found no difference in decay between fluoridated and non-fluoridated communities.[4] Even now in Western Europe, 97% of the countries have chosen fluoride-free water.

Take Matters Into Your Own Clean Hands

Chlorine and fluoride have also been known to displace iodine from the body. Iodine is an essential mineral required for proper thyroid hormone function. As mentioned, toxic heavy metals like small amounts of lead or arsenic or mercury can also be present in your water. These poisons can suppress the functioning of your glands. Isn't it coincidental that thyroid disorders have been on the rise as chlorine, fluoride, heavy metals, and other chemical toxins have become more prevalent in our environment? Consider these contaminants in addition to animal manures, chemical fertilizers and other agricultural wastes as well as the dozens of toxic chemicals with which industry pollutes the sky and the rivers. Do you want to put that junk into your body?

To avoid this potential source of toxic contamination, I recommend to my patients that they drink filtered water. This can be anything from distilled water or water treated by reverse osmosis, to plain old simple and cheap carbon filtration. Any filtration method that decreases the amount of contamination is better than drinking chemically polluted water. It is preferable to have a water filter in your home so that you can avoid buying water in plastic bottles. Water stored in plastic is not healthful, as you'll read below, and also contributes to landfill waste.

For my patients I recommend AquaLiv™ water purification systems that remove microorganisms, heavy metals, chemical toxins including chlorine byproducts, and even fluoride. I am advocating this particular filter because it not only removes physical contaminants, it also clears the electromagnetic contaminants of the water. Just like in Nature, these filters vortex the water which cleanses it of any past memory. This is about as close to having a natural spring percolating clean energized water into your glass as it gets. Please see how you can acquire an AquaLiv™ filter that gives you Nature's water at the end of the book (see Sources). The company is offering a discount to Nature's Diet readers.

Your Number is UP

Buying water stored in plastic bottles is not recommended. Even safe plastic can leach chemicals into the water. Also, the amount of waste generated from plastic water bottles can be overwhelming for our planet. Just travel around the world a bit and you'll notice developing countries do not recycle as evidenced from the incredible number of plastic bags and bottles along the roads. One world is all we have and we all share it together. We may not share the same land but we do share the same water and the same air. The actions of one people can and does affect the natural resources we all share.

Monitor your water intake by drinking from a safe type of water bottle. This makes it easier to identify how much you drink in a day. The best water bottle containers are made from glass or stainless steel because they do not leach chemicals into the water. An old quart jar or juice bottle serves well. If your water bottle is plastic turn it over and look at the bottom. Make sure it does not have the numbers 3, 6, or 7, which are now considered to leak poisonous chemicals such as PVC, Polystyrene, and BPA, which are toxic and which can interfere with hormone levels.

If you must use a plastic bottle, choose one with the numbers 2, 4, or 5 on the bottom. If it has the number "1", then it is safe for only one use, and even then you should be careful, because in fact, there really are **no** safe plastics. Even the so called "safe plastics" can leach into whatever liquid is being stored in them. Anything, especially water stored in plastic bottles, should be kept away from the light or the heat, and especially out of the sunlight sitting in your car all day.

Wise Water Tips

For a person who is generally healthy with no major health problems, he or she can start by drinking water in the quantity of approximately half their body weight in ounces of water. For instance, if you weigh 100 pounds you would sip 50 ounces during the day. Recognize the word is sip, not gulp! This does not mean that you are to drink eight glasses of water a day! Your body has numerous mechanisms continually monitoring your chemistry and which are making sure you don't have too much or too little water. If a full glass of water is drunk all at once, these mechanisms will kick in and yes… the pee-pee dance it will be! *The key is sipping water little by little all day long, not gulping down a glass at a time!* Think of it as an IV drip-drip-dripping into your gut instead of into your arm.

At first, it may be difficult to drink this quantity of water… especially because when the body is not accustomed to this amount, the "need to pee" will be turned up. This is not a bad thing either because the extra water is releasing wastes which are stored in the tissues and cleaning the entire urinary system as it exits. It will take about a week but soon enough the number of trips to the bathroom will decrease significantly. This is because your body is becoming used to the extra water intake and is beginning to utilize it by absorbing more of the fluid.

Think of your cells as pieces of dehydrated fruit. Something dried out will not completely hydrate if it is just dipped in and out of water a few times. A shriveled old prune needs to be soaked in water overnight to regain its moisture content. In the same way, your cells need to have constant soaking over a period of time. This is why it is SO IMPORTANT to sip on small amounts of water all day to become rehydrated.

The only time the sipping rule doesn't apply is when you are very thirsty and your body is already craving water from dehydration. Of course this is an appropriate time to gulp until you are satisfied. This also would not apply to the moment you first wake up in the morning. After sleeping eight hours without drinking, the body is in need of fluid. So, the moment you open your eyes and sit up in bed, reach over to your night stand and gulp down a full glass of water. This will act as a flush and wash out the wastes that your body accumulated during your rest.

A few more water drinking tips… (who'd ever think that drinking water could have so many requirements?) As mentioned, sipping and not gulping is important. So is not drinking water within a half hour of a meal. So many of my patients look at me in disbelief, "What Doc? I can't believe that! The only time I ever drink water is with my meals!" I tell them if they drink too much water with their meals, it is likely to dilute their natural enzymes and acid reserves. These enzymes and hydrochloric acid need to be at full strength to digest food completely. How can the acid in your gut turn that chunk of roast beef into a liquid soup if you just dumped in a bunch of water and the acid now is weaker and more diluted?

The Pee Pee Dance

I have also found that patients get better rest if they discontinue drinking water an hour or two before going to bed. This is especially important for men who need to get up frequently due to an enlarged prostate. Giving the body a full two hours without fluids before sleep can make a real difference for those needing a full night's sleep without getting up to urinate. If you find your body is really not used to the change in hydration and you are urinating all the time, then you may need to allow 3-4 hours before bed to stop drinking water.

Speaking of the prostate, I know some of you suffer greatly with frequent urination due to prostate inflammation, irritable bladder, or persistent bladder infections. Drinking more water is the last thing you feel like doing because you already have to constantly go to the bathroom. In reality, it is the most important for your health. Again, you have to think of how effectively water puts out the fires of inflammation. I have been impressed clinically by those patients who have complained of urinary inflammation and frequency of urination, and who have actually improved their ability to hold their urine by drinking more water.

The explanation for this is several-fold. First, when urine is not diluted with water it is more concentrated in acid, salts, and waste products which makes it more inflammatory. These wastes are hot and burning. They have a pro-inflammatory action on the organs through which the urine passes: the kidneys, bladder, prostate, urethra and vaginal areas. Simply diluting this urine with more water lessens the irritation of these organs as it discharges the wastes. This gives these tissues a chance to heal. This is especially good news for those with chronic or persistent urinary infections and tendencies to yeast or bacterial infections. Second, increasing the volume of urine being eliminated acts as a washing of the organs. Think of an increased urinary flow like the water from a hose washing the mud off the car. In this case "the mud" is the bacteria or other bad microorganisms and the waste they feed on. Thirdly, just running more water through the urinary system exercises those smooth muscles and strengthens them. Stronger muscles means better urine control.

Too Hot, Too Cold, and Just Right

It is best if water is drunk at room temperature, body temperature, or even warmer unless you are overheated. Hot water is higher in thermal energy and when ingested the heat disperses throughout the body adding a greater amount of kinetic energy[5] to your system. Cold water on the other hand will absorb thermal energy or heat which means it robs energy from your body.

Ice cold water or even cold water can shock the metabolic functions of the body and put more stress on the hormone systems of the adrenals and thyroid glands. Cold temperatures push blood away and warm temperatures attract blood which improves circulation giving a reddish glow. If you drink ice cold water you will be pushing blood away from the stomach which only decreases digestive function.

If your body is already in an overheated state, cool water can be helpful in dispersing the heat. If you are on the cooler side however, ice cold water lowers the body's core temperature so it requires your own kinetic energy to warm it back up to 98.6 degrees. That is hard work! Remember, your body likes to conserve energy and take the path of least resistance just like you- don't be so hard on it! Give it a lazy-boy day once in a while.

Although ice is an element provided by Nature, it is not something that our ancestors living in mild temperatures encountered often. Iceboxes are a relatively new discovery by humans since their use has only become popularized since the mid-nineteenth century. Your genes have only had a couple hundred years to adapt to food made cold by mechanical refrigeration. Our ancient ancestors didn't have iceboxes or refrigerators or freezers so ice cream, Slurpies, and iced lemonade martinis were out of the question while they were roaming the countryside. (I'm sure though they would have enjoyed 31 Flavors, or a Happy Hour once in a while considering the challenges they endured!)

If you are someone who has great difficulty drinking plain water because of its tastelessness, non-caffeinated herbal teas or a squeeze of fresh lemon to clean filtered water are both great options. For some people who really have trouble getting it down, it is also possible to take 100% fruit juice and split it 50/50 with purified water in the beginning. As the body gets accustomed to this taste you can dilute the juice further by adding more plain water until eventually the juice is completely eliminated. Even plain carbonated water is better than drinking fluids that are filled with sugar and artificial flavors and colors, such as soda pops, artificial juices, and sport drinks. Adding a little lemon or lime to carbonated water is a great beverage alternative to drinking a soda pop when you are in social environments.

Happy drinking and happy peeing! It is a good thing!

---

[1]Path of least resistance: the route objects moving through a system will take.

[2]Resonance: the system oscillates distinctly at particular frequencies. The system is able to store and transfer energy between storage modes (in this case water to human). Resonance phenomena occur with all types of vibrations or waves: there is mechanical resonance, acoustic resonance, electromagnetic resonance, and resonance of quantum wave functions.

[3]Rocha-Amador D, et al. (2007). Decreased intelligence in children and exposure to fluoride and arsenic in drinking water. Cadernos de Saude Publica 23(Suppl 4):S579-87

[4]www.fluoridealert.org/fluoride-facts.htm

[5]thermal energy: the total of the kinetic energy due to the motion of particles and the potential energy associated with the vibrational and electrical energy of atoms. Temperature is a measure of kinetic energy. The faster the particles the more energy created and the higher the temperature. Heat moves from higher temperature areas to lower temperature areas. In this example, heat moves into cold water from the body.

START TODAY:

- Figure the amount of water you are to consume by taking your total body weight and divide by two. This will give you the number of ounces of water you should consume. If you weigh 100 pounds then 100/2= 50 ounces.

- Choose water which is purified through filtration. (see Sources) You will start off the day by rolling out of bed and drinking one full glass of water on rising. This is the only glass you gulp down at once. The rest of the day just take sips of water all day long. Monitor your water intake by carrying around a "safe" water bottle so you can be sure you are getting the appropriate amounts.

- Drink no water within half an hour of your meals and make sure you are not drinking within a couple hours of bedtime.

- Choose to drink only room-temperature water unless you are overheated or cold. In these cases you can drink cooled or heated water.

- Non-caffeinated herbal teas, extra-diluted fruit juice, and squeezing fresh lemon or lime into purified water or carbonated water are other options to add variety and are especially helpful for those who don't like the taste of water plain.

Summary: This is what I'm doing up to this point, each day adds onto the next

Day 1: Food awareness: Keep a diary of my foods. I am accountable.

Day 2: Water: Sip half my body weight in ounces throughout the day.

Day 3
Movement

Alright! You made it through the second day! How is it going? Peeing a lot yet? Good! If you don't use it you lose it and getting those kidneys to function is a very beneficial and healthy practice. In that same sense having water run through the system is cleansing for those prone to infections.

Today we are going to further boost oxygen and circulation. A dear friend and mentor of mine, who was an osteopathic physician, reminded his patients that "Circulation is Life and Stagnation is Death." There is so much truth to this. We are circulating beings and circulation is absolutely essential to every single cell to bring oxygen, water, and nutrients and carry away the wastes and toxins. As the heart pumps, the blood is pumped and freely circulates through the blood vessels if they are healthy and not filled with atherosclerotic plaques. One of the best ways to keep the heart healthy is to have a healthy work out and today you are going to give it one! You must move that body daily, and this is the start of day two.

The "E" word is the other cuss word you know as "Exercise." It can be a real challenge for so many because it usually represents something that is painful and hard work. It really doesn't need to be, though. Really, exercise can be any activity that gets your heart and breath and blood moving for a period of time. Hiking counts, dancing counts, golfing too, if you are quickly walking from hole to hole, bicycling, swimming, team sports, and yes, sex counts too!

As the body increases physical movement, the heart pumps more frequently and forcefully. This force propels oxygen-filled blood throughout the body. During the movement the body also breathes more which further increases oxygen levels and exhales the waste carbon dioxide. Oxygen is the source of life, without it you couldn't live but 3-5 minutes. (The author resumes no responsibility if you try holding your breath this long to see if this is actually true.) Exercise increases circulation which then fills the blood and your cells with this life-giving oxygen.

Moving the body with exercise and other activities is a very effective way to eliminate toxins which have built up in the body. These are toxins our body naturally makes as well as those with which we come in contact in our environment. Every day, we are exposed to heavy metals, chemical fumes, and toxic residues from thousands of sources. Vigorously exhaling carbon dioxide is one method the body utilizes to get rid of these toxic wastes. The breath can even expel heavy metals like lead and mercury and arsenic!

Exercise will also raise your temperature causing you to sweat. This is another method of removing toxins from the body through the skin. Each of your cells is also excreting waste as a substance called lymphatic fluid. This fluid is only able to be eliminated from the body if the muscles contract and push it through the body. Therefore movement, especially vigorous exercise, helps the body remove lymphatic waste from your lymph glands, organs, tissues and skin, as well.

In Nature, animals move their bodies all day in search of food. Their muscles are contracting and forcing the waste out of their cells into the blood to be eliminated. Our ancestors also spent much time moving their bodies searching for food or tending their land. Today, most of us do not have the types of jobs that allow us to replicate what Nature intended. We miss the opportunity to move our bodies because we sit most of the day doing our jobs. To compensate for this lack of activity we need to get our bodies moving whether outside on the sidewalks, in organized workout routines, or invigorating activities.

Invigorate the Body

So today…building upon the water sipping from yesterday…you must get the body moving! It really doesn't matter what it is - just move! It can be as simple as walking through your neighborhood or on trails with your doggie, or taking up that dance class so you could be like one of the "stars" you watch on TV (without the judging, of course), or as complex as doing a synchronized step-aerobics or kick-boxing. Some other ideas are bicycling, swimming, jumping rope, walking up hills, bouncing on a trampoline rebounder, hiking, horseback riding, etc., you name it. The activity itself isn't what it important. What is important is that you just do something to get the body moving, the blood pumping, and the air in your lungs ventilating.

Getting outside in the fresh air away from busy streets is a nice option instead of being inside a gym breathing the air of 30 people on treadmills in a closed room. Brisk walking, especially if there are some good hills involved, is an excellent way to get the body circulation moving. It really doesn't have to be a long walk. Thirty minutes is all you really need on a daily basis to get the blood moving.

As with your diet diary, you will want to create structure in your exercise program as well. Whether that is with a trainer in the gym or on your own, there should be some level of organization to keep track of your improvement. One way to gain structure is by utilizing an exercise journal. Simply write down your daily activity and a measurement of what you did. You may choose to write down the distance you walked or ran and you may also choose to write the time it took you to go that distance. If you are lifting weights, you may choose to record the amount of weight that is being lifted and the number of times you lifted it.

Why is this important? This will allow you to push yourself to improve your scores from the day before. This helps you to remain accountable and to continually push yourself that extra bit to make sure you stay on the edge of success. One method you may choose to do this is to set out a marked distance and time it. Each day, you'll want to improve your time from the previous day even if it is just one second each day. That stopwatch is your own personal trainer and it is able to make you more accountable. Just remember… write it down!

Sometimes you may be pressed for time and not have a full 30 minutes to dedicate to movement. It is not the amount of time or the length of distance which is most important for the benefits of exercise. It is about getting the heart to pump and the blood to MOVE! If you know you don't have enough time to have a complete workout, just do something simple to get the heart and lungs to pump and oxygenate.

Here is an example of an activity you may choose to do if you are short on time. It is quick but invigorating. Choose a hill and run up the hill as fast and as hard as you can for about 10-20 seconds. Pretend you are running for your life! Pretend you are running from a natural disaster, from a hungry tiger, or - from your ex-spouse! Then, let the body recuperate as you walk back down the hill. Repeat this a few sets if you have the time. This is an effective way to get that blood to pump and the oxygen to ventilate even if you are short on time.

Ask yourself too; what is the purpose of this movement? What is my purpose for exercising? For some it might be just to get into the healthy habit, for others it may be to lose weight, for others maybe it's a stress reducer. All of them are good reasons to move the body. The intensity of the movement will have to be more intense if you are doing it for weight loss and less intense if it is just to get refocused after a long day.

Many of you know not to exercise soon after eating. Don't eat just before exercising but rather allow an hour or two for your food to digest after eating. A light snack of fruit or a healthy smoothie is acceptable up to 20 minutes before exercising. Also make sure that you do not exercise within a couple hours of going to sleep. Exercising is stimulating to the body and can make it difficult to get into a restful state. Try exercising in the morning or after work when you need an energetic pick-me-up.

START TODAY:

- Put at least 30 minutes aside each day for movement activity. Make sure you do not exercise within a couple hours after eating. Don't exercise in the evenings before bed.

- To keep yourself accountable, along with your food journal, keep detailed notes about your movement. Record at least one of multiple factors so you can see your progress. You may record the distance you went, the minutes it took, the quantity of repetitions or the amount you may have lifted. This will be the foundation to track your improvement over time. It will also be helpful for your coach to see if you are making progress in your personal program.

Get the body moving, get it circulating, and start to witness the results which are about to unfold!

Summary: This is what I'm doing up to this point, each day adds onto the next

Day 1: Food awareness: Keep a diary of my foods. I am accountable.

Day 2: Water: Sip half my body weight in ounces throughout the day.

Day 3: Movement: Some exercise performed every day. Note it in my diary.

Day 4
Regular Meals

So now, on to the food! One of the most common misunderstandings I hear from my patients is, "Maybe if I just stop eating a couple meals a day I will lose this extra weight." This couldn't be farther from the truth. The mistake most people make is thinking they are doing themselves a benefit by skipping meals. They think that eating no food will somehow equal less weight on their body. Sure, starvation will sooner or later cause you to lose weight, but what happens when you return to eating? All the weight comes back!

As in Nature, a fire requires a steady source of fuel to keep burning. Putting too large a log on a small fire will cause it to smolder and will snuff it out! Think of this weak fire as your "metabolic digestive fire" and that large log as a big fat meal. You can see that if you eat nothing all morning, and sometimes even skip lunch, your metabolic fire remains quiet and low. By the end of the day you are so hungry that you eat a big meal. That is one big log your metabolic fires are unable to burn completely because they are so weak. This can lead to undigested food and inefficient metabolism which means inability to lose weight.

Also realize that when you do not eat for an extended period of time, your body will scream out, "HEY I AM STARVING HERE!"

This sends chemical messages to your brain and body, preparing them for what could be the next great depression. The body sends a clear chemical signal to all the cells: "SAVE!" If this happens, the body instinctively turns down its metabolic fires and burns less fat to energy. It will actually conserve your body fat just in case it doesn't see food for a while. When you do eat again, it says, "HEY, THANKS A LOT, IN CASE THIS STARVING THING HAPPENS AGAIN, I'M GOING TO STORE SOME OF THIS FOOD FOR NEXT TIME." Sure enough, what ends up happening is you actually have more difficulty losing weight in the future because the body is protecting you from future starvation.

So think about what you are doing the next time you go all day without eating. Maybe you are the type who is so busy at work that you have no time to eat all day. Maybe you are the type who comes home eight hours later and you are jittery because of low blood sugar or maybe you just lived on coffee, Coke™, or candy (the infamous 3 Cs!) By dinnertime, you are ready to FEAST on half a cow. And because you feast when the digestive fires are quiet, it is just like throwing that big log on that teeny tiny fire: Woopff! The fire gets snuffed out! This simply magnifies your already poor digestion and you end up with bloating, heartburn, belching, and passing gas (This might be fun for some of you, not for most, especially those who are the recipients of your fetid fumes!)

As opposed to skipping meals on a daily basis, strict water fasting under the discretion of a health minded practitioner can be very beneficial. A therapeutic water fast can have a profound impact on chronic conditions and overall health. I have been amazed witnessing healing miracles when fasting patients both under my supervision and at fasting clinics. Fasting can promote healing, especially during acute illness. Starve a fever <u>and</u> starve a cold. Have you seen what an animal does when it is sick? That's right! It fasts so its body can focus on healing, not digesting. Please see "Sources" for clinics specializing in therapeutic fasting and do not fast without supervision.

The focus for this fourth day is not to be concerned about what you are eating quite yet. Rather, your focus today is to have at the minimum three moderately-sized meals, or if you need to eat more often, take these three meals and cut them in half and eat a total of 6 times a day about every 2-3 hours. Again, it does not matter what you are eating right now, just practice getting the fires stoked and the body heated up ready to burn!

There are a couple dos and don'ts here as far as timing is concerned. Try to eat the meals about the same time day after day. This scheduling gets the body into a rhythm which is going to be very important when we talk about sleep. Speaking of sleep, allow your body at least three hours before going to sleep after eating. We want the body to have the food liquefied and ready to absorb its goodness before you rest your head. While you sleep, you want the body to go into cleaning mode, not digesting food mode. This is to ensure that the body rhythm is maintained.

START TODAY:

- Eat 3 moderately-sized meals for breakfast, lunch and dinner, or eat 6 smaller meals about every 2 hours.

- Eat about the same time each day and stick to this schedule for the rest of the program.

- Do not eat before going to bed or before heavy activity.

Summary: This is what I'm doing up to this point, each day adds onto the next

Day 1: Food awareness: Keep a diary of my foods. I am accountable.

Day 2: Water: Sip half my body weight in ounces throughout the day.

Day 3: Movement: Some exercise performed every day. Note it in my diary.

Day 4: Regular meals: Eat about the same time each day.

Day 5
Vegetables & Living Foods

Over the years, my clinical practice has taught me that there are three main factors which will most affect a person's health. If a patient is dedicated and consistent in these three areas, they are putting themselves on the path toward optimal health. From these clinical observations, I came up with the idea of the 50-50-50 rule.

The first 50 represents the consumption of 50% of your body weight in ounces of water which you have already started. The second 50, which you have also started, is moving the body in some form of activity at least 50% of the days of the week. In this program, though, instead of 3-4 days a week you are exercising every single day. Finally, the third and most important component is including 50% of your diet in vegetable material. Yes, you heard correctly and I will repeat it: One half the weight of your entire food intake should be VEGETABLES!! The Jolly Green Giant will be proud!

So what is the big deal with veggies? Why such a massive load? One reason is that vegetables are made of natural fibers that give them strength, crispness and texture. When that same fiber is chewed and swallowed, it acts like a net of sponges which prevent the not-so-good things in your diet from being absorbed.

This is especially good if this meal is rich in sugar, starch, fat or grease because the vegetable fiber will prevent these from being absorbed into the body easily. The more fiber there is, the more space it occupies in your intestines, which means the less bad stuff can be absorbed directly. So your nummy rich pasta with cream sauce and the crème brulee for dessert will get trapped in the fibers of the vegetables you ate, which slows or prevents the absorption of these rich fatty and sugary foods. Of course this is extra important if you are prone to high blood sugar or if you want to lower your cholesterol or if you want to just lose more weight.

This little trick is like cheating the system! Really! Think about it: what happens in your gut if you eat pepperoni pizza and pair it with a soda pop? All the grease and sugar and all the artificial flavorings, chemical seasonings, and additives would have 100% contact with the inner walls of your intestines. The more contact this food has with the intestinal wall, the greater the amount and the faster the speed with which it will be absorbed into the blood stream. This high amount of fat and sugar is more than the body can deal with at one time. Such an increase in the blood will trigger the pancreas to dump insulin. More on insulin in a minute.

Now take that same amount of pizza and soda and pair it with a huge plate of salad or even just raw veggies so you are eating 50% pizza/soda and 50% veggies. A bite of pizza, a bite of veggies, a sip of soda, a bite of pizza, a bite of veggies and what is created is a mixture of pizza-veggie goop! (Remember, however, that the veggies are going to equal the weight of the pizza and the pop.) But this time, much less sugar or grease comes in contact with the lining of your intestines. Why? Well, because there is more space occupied by vegetable fiber which contains no sugar or grease. It literally acts as a space filler to prevent the fat or sugar from being absorbed! The beauty is that vegetable fiber will not increase your blood sugar, your cholesterol, or your weight; in fact, it will balance all three.

Vegetable Imposters

Not all vegetables are created equally, and many people are justly confused as to what a vegetable really is. First, it is important to clarify which foods are often thought of as vegetables but which are actually vegetable imposters. When I ask my patients to devote

50% of each plate to vegetables they may say something like, "Oh, that should be easy, Doctor. My family just loves baked potatoes or corn on the cob." Many think of corn and potatoes as members of the vegetable group. In this case they do not get honored with such a noble title; both of these foods are classified as starches or carbohydrates rather than vegetables.

What is a starch? Starch is a carbohydrate composed of glucose sugars stacked up together. It is very important to understand this because when starch is broken down in the body it turns back into pure glucose. It is true that our body needs glucose; it is very important to keep our brains functioning on all cylinders. But when we have an excess amount of this sugar, the body stores it as fat. This is considered to be the primary cause of the health problems among Americans and the populations of other Westernized countries.

When sugar is ingested into the body, the pancreas responds by secreting insulin. Insulin's job is to push the sugar into the cells so it can be used. If there is excess sugar, the pancreas secretes even more insulin. Insulin is a storage molecule. If insulin goes high, it sends a message to the body to STORE! (Usually in those places you are trying to make it go away!) If it can push no more sugar into your cells then it will begin to make fat with the excess sugar. At the same time it will prevent any fat in your storage (spare tires) from being burned and converted back into energy.

We love our sugar and starch and consume more than our bodies need on a daily basis. Eventually, this diet of high-energy carbohydrates causes insulin to be secreted in such high amounts that your tissues no longer respond to it. This is called insulin resistance and it often leads to type-2 diabetes and metabolic syndrome. Metabolic syndrome is the condition of having high blood sugar, high lipids (cholesterol and triglycerides) and high blood pressure. It is a risk factor for diabetes mellitus and coronary artery disease.

So, corn is not going to be labeled as a vegetable and neither are potatoes. They are both foods dense in starch, which means the body will break them down into glucose sugar. If they are eaten in excess, you will gain weight because they will cause your sugar levels to increase, your insulin to increase, and the message to your body will be: STORE FAT!

All vegetables dug from the soil, such as potatoes, sweet potatoes, yams, carrots, beets, parsnips, turnips, rutabagas, and yucca are also high in starch. The part we eat is the root of the plant; the part which sends green stems and leaves through the soil up to the sun. Roots are high in starch because they provide the plant with the energy it needs to sprout from the darkness and grow into the light. Because these vegetables harvested from the ground are high in starch, they will not be considered a part of the 50% vegetables UNLESS they are RAW!

Let's make one more exclusion here since your bubble has already been burst from the potato and corn thing. Green peas are a legume, actually a member of the dried bean family rather than a vegetable. Dried beans (not green beans) are predominantly a starch and are not considered a vegetable or a protein substitute as is commonly thought. Beans and legumes are mostly starch so green peas will also be considered a starch rather than a vegetable. So yes, Forest and Jenny fit like peas and carrots because they are both starches when cooked! Peas are not to be used as part of the 50% vegetable requirement unless they are raw or still in their pods.

A Raw Deal

Yes raw! Why you may ask? Well, the title of this book is *"Nature's Diet"* and in keeping with the theme of the book we have to look back to Nature. Now, where in any part of this world have you ever seen an animal with a wok busily stir-frying their vegetables? How's that for a visual? So, shouldn't we ask then, if the cooking of food was an essential for life, wouldn't the animals be doing it?

Humans have an intelligence that surpasses all the creatures that have ever evolved on this planet. We differ from the animals in that we have a sophisticated brain and a developed frontal lobe which allows us to plan, make decisions and think constructively and creatively. Because of this, we have used our ability to make and use tools, harness fire and modernize our lives. It is through our intelligence that we have not only advanced our state of living, but have also forgotten our natural ways of the past.

Our primitive ancestors used intuition and instinct to help them survive difficult conditions. They are an excellent example to emulate and our best present day resource on to how humans can live in alignment with Nature. Of course hit movies like "Avatar" although fantasy, clearly demonstrate the benefits of living in harmony with Nature. The primitive people on Pandora seemed to enjoy the same conveniences of technological man without scientific gadgets or the destruction of their resources. They were completely sustained, nourished, and nurtured by following Nature's path.

Wild animals eat only food that has been raw and or decomposing. Primates whose digestive system is the most similar to ours eat no cooked foods in the wild. Primitive humans, however, were the only animals who harnessed fire for warmth and cooking. We have done so for millennia even though fire has only been harnessed for a mere fraction of time when compared to all of human existence. It is estimated that early humans subsisted on raw foods for almost 100,000 generations before regularly utilizing fire to cook food.[1] Having a logical thinking brain has allowed us to make use of fire in ways that animals do not and provide more options for food that are not available to other creatures.

Because of this, humans have been eating cooked foods since primitive times and we need not adopt a completely raw food approach. The ancient human diet was predominantly raw sources with some cooked foods. We want to mirror Nature here and use an abundance of raw foods without going completely fanatical and discontinuing the use of cooked food our ancestors discovered.

YIN YANG

Cooking has both its drawbacks and benefits. When food is cooked, heat changes the molecules so that the body can break it down more easily. Think what fire does to anything if it is heated long enough; it turns it back into ashes. Heat takes a complex molecule like starch or protein and breaks it down into small parts like glucose and amino acids and makes it easier to assimilate. This way one can eat less food and get more nutrients out of it.

Some people who eat only raw vegetables have a hard time maintaining enough weight because their food is only partially digested; cooking can therefore be beneficial particularly for those people who have poor digestion. Cooking actually breaks down the large complex molecules of the plant making it easier to digest.

Starch molecules are broken down into smaller carbohydrates chains making them more easily absorbed. Since we don't have four stomachs to aid in digestion of raw plants like a cow does, cooking is helpful to break down the nutrition locked in the dense cellulose fiber in plants. Cooked foods are better for people who are nutritionally deficient, underweight, and having difficulty digesting food because of diarrhea or other intestinal aggravations.

In fact, if you are someone who suffers from indigestion and gas consider eating only steamed vegetables or vegetables cooked in soups. In addition to eating no raw vegetables, also avoid vegetables high in sulfur such as broccoli, cabbage, cauliflower, Brussels sprouts, kale, collards, onions, garlic, and peppers. These vegetables can be especially gassy if they are raw, but also may cause gas in a sensitive person even if they are cooked. If you have digestive complaints you should also avoid fruit products until you are feeling better. It is especially important not to eat any fruit during your meals; more on that later. Remember not to drink water with your meals and chew your food slowly and intentionally until it is a liquid in your mouth. If digestion is really a problem you may also consider adding a supplement such as digestive enzymes, papaya chewable enzymes, hydrochloric acid, or even activated charcoal for excess gas and bloating. Long term maintenance of the digestive tract is benefitted by taking probiotic beneficial bacteria. These subjects will be discussed shortly.

Also worth noting is that Chinese Medicine classifies raw vegetables as being very YIN. This is the opposite of YANG. What this means is that these YIN vegetables are cooling and will make a body cooler or more YIN when they are consumed. This is a great idea for someone who is on the hotter YANG side because his or her body is on fire due to inflammation. They may even appear red and hot in the face. YANG dominant people also tend to have higher blood pressure, higher cholesterol, higher blood sugar, or are overweight. Heavy doses of raw vegetables may not be a good choice for you if you are someone who is cold all the time, underweight, have low blood pressure, or if you live in a cold climate. If this sounds like you, then your YIN qualities are too strong and you should cut back on the total amount of raw veggies and consume mostly steamed, stir-fried, or cooked veggies in soups.

Cooking can also break down some chemicals in plants that can serve to block nutrient absorption. Phytates are present in many grains and beans and unless they are soaked, cooked, or sprouted, can inhibit the absorption of important minerals. Minerals themselves are not destroyed with cooking. They can be lost though if you boil your vegetables in water and then dump the nutrient-filled water down the sink. We will discuss this more in the section on food preparation but boiling vegetables is not a good idea unless you are making a soup and drinking the nutrient-dense broth too.

In general, heat can destroy vital nutrients in your raw food such as enzymes and co-enzymes which we know as vitamins. However, some nutrients like beta carotene, an anti-cancer antioxidant found in orange colored foods like carrots and sweet potatoes and squash, is actually better absorbed if the food is cooked. If food is cooked at high heat for long periods of time though, such as in canning, the beta carotene is transformed into a molecule that cannot be used by the body. High heat can also transform proteins and fats in your food into harmful substances which have been known to cause cancer and other diseases. This will be discussed in later days when we talk about protein and fat.

Little packets of LIGHT

Nature provides food to us in a living form. The moment a plant is plucked from the vine, it no longer has the capacity to regenerate the nutrients it did while alive. Therefore, the food we purchase in the grocery store is already beginning the process of decay: returning to dust. Nature's decay mechanisms are acting on it as air and light and microorganisms begin to break down produce *the moment it is picked*. When a plant is harvested, electrical ions are released and the energetic qualities of plants decrease. The longer it is in storage, the more the energy decreases. Living foods are more vital and nutrient dense because they are actively living. The sooner you can eat them after they are harvested, the better. Vitamins are destroyed not only by heat but also by exposure to air and light as well. Try to buy your produce from farmer's markets or ask your grocer which days their produce shipments come in so you can take full advantage of their freshness.

Live food is activated food! Your cells are alive so doesn't it just make sense to give your cells more of what they already are? It makes real sense to feed your cells with food that is loaded with the qualities of life. Feed your body with biologically activated minerals, vitamins, enzymes, DNA and RNA, and dozens of other activated proteins that are found only in food that is alive. Sprouts of any type are excellent food that is full of activated living nutrition because sprouts are still alive when you eat them! Think of a grain or a seed as being asleep; all its metabolic processes are quiet. Add a little water to this guy and voila! The seed becomes quickened with life and all the cellular components become activated as ATP energy is being made from the chlorophyll and sunlight through photosynthesis. This plant is now alive and filled with living energy!

We are all energetic electric beings. Even rocks and dirt have energy which is composed of the electrical charges of their constituent protons and electrons. We all literally run on energy that has been transmuted in one way or another from the energy of the sun. The First Law of Thermodynamics is clear. It states energy is neither created nor destroyed but just changes form. Nature will conserve energy by transforming the energy or change it from one form to another. For this reason, this scientific law has also been called The Law of the Conservation of Energy.

Little packets of light energy from the sun called photons are stored in plants. These biophotons, or energy packets, are then passed on to us when we eat these plants. There is some idea that these biophotons contain vibrational information which is vital to insuring that our cells stay in the proper frequency with the earth and sun. The greater the biophoton concentration, the greater the vital energy that a particular plant or animal provides. The more light a food is able to store, the more energetic it is for our bodies. Freshly grown organic vegetables and fruits which have been allowed to sun-ripen on the vine are rich in light energy. Compare the amount of photon energy available in a dried seed compared to a seed that has been sprouted and reaches for the light.

We live not on our food but rather on the energy that our food provides. Additionally, you could say we do not simply make energy from the food we eat but we also assimilate the energy of *the energy of the food* (biophotons) we eat. It took a long time for me to understand what my teacher was trying to tell me that first day we met. Our body not only lives off the energy it makes from food but the energy the food has captured from the sun and gives us directly. This energy frequency flows through plants and is passed on as a living spark for our cells. This highlights the law of thermodynamics, as the energy is just passed from one being to the next to the next. The more biophoton energy from the sun has been captured in your food the more activated nutrients will be passed onto your cells. This is the basis of an entirely separate subject applying quantum physics and the frequencies of minerals and vitamins and the field of homeopathy and radionics.

"It's Alive! It's Alive"

Raw foods as found in Nature have multiple health-endowing qualities. Eating something which is alive and fresh provides vitamins and enzymes which are not always present in food that has been cooked or preserved. Realistically speaking, however, our busy lives make it nearly impossible for every man to have a garden and pick food from the vine and eat it on the spot. We are dependent on convenience and simple preparations. Nature's path is clearly laid out for us, but in this day, we have to do our best, and we aren't always going to be 100% compliant.

You may have heard that a primary benefit of eating foods raw is that they provide an abundance of enzymes which can aid digestion and detoxification. These living, activated enzymes found in raw foods are destroyed in the cooking process. Although certainly beneficial, the relatively small amount of these enzymes may not help with the digestion of the foods themselves. In fact, there is still little evidence that the enzymes present in raw food have a huge impact on human health. Regardless of this, Nature requires these enzymes to help the fruits to ripen and the seeds to sprout. Whether or not they serve a vital role for the animals or humans who ingest them is still debatable.

Ideally, it would be best to eat the majority of our food from Nature raw and unprocessed. This is especially wise for those people who have strong YANG qualities or those whose levels of triglycerides, cholesterol, and sugar are elevated. Remember that vegetable cellulose fibers trap the excess fat and sugar in your diet but to do this effectively you want to consume about 80% of your total vegetable intake as raw vegetables. So of the 50% of the total weight of your vegetable intake, the majority (80%) should be RAW. You can even eat more than 50% of your total intake if you wish to; in fact eat your heart out! Eat as many vegetables as you wish! Go ahead, cram yourself full!

Animals like cows and gorillas, that consume large amounts of raw plant material, need to eat all day long to get enough calories to satisfy their needs. This is in contrast to carnivores like lions and tigers who can manage with a few meals each week because their meals are high in fat and protein. When you begin to change your foods to include higher amounts of vegetables and plant-based foods, you may find that you are hungrier more often. This is typical because there are fewer calories provided by vegetables. This means you will need to eat more vegetables at your meal and even between your meals to keep you satisfied. Go ahead and eat like a cow! Your hunger craving is normal and you can follow it by eating these vegetables through the day if you need to.

They will not cause problems with weight because vegetables are very low in calories and not as concentrated as other foods. A pound of lettuce has about 60 calories while a pound of potatoes has about 420 calories. What a difference a pound makes! Could you eat 7 pounds of lettuce??? Basically vegetables are so cool because you can eat so many of them and they will not affect you negatively!

So for today here is the task: go ahead and eat whatever you wish to eat... sure! "Even a Big Mac?" Sure! Whatever you wish! Here is the catch, match it with an equal weighted amount of vegetables from the list below. Vegetables need to count for at least one half the weight of all the food that is consumed at that meal.

Now some of you must be wondering about breakfast by now. Well, let us just for now continue eating the breakfast that you are used to, whatever it may be. We will get to the breakfast options coming up soon.

---

[1]There's no evidence for the regular, controlled use of fire for cooking until 300k-400k years ago. For around 1.6 million years (almost 100,000 generations), our ancestors were eating meat without cooking it. (Apr 2009). "Fire in the Earth System". Science 324 (5926): 481

START TODAY:

- Eat like a cow! Eat vegetables all day long if you need to. Remember vegetables have fewer calories so you will probably need to eat plenty of them and eat them often throughout the day to keep you satisfied. Make sure at least 50% of the weight of your meal is in vegetables, and preferably at least 80% of those vegetables are raw. The other 20% can be eaten lightly steamed or stir fried or in soups. We'll talk about food preparation in a later chapter.

- If you are someone who has digestive difficulty with raw foods, eat only cooked vegetables for right now. If you are someone who runs cold or if you are in the middle of winter or living in a cold climate, you may also choose to eat mostly cooked vegetables.

Summary: This is what I'm doing up to this point, each day adds onto the next

Day 1: Food awareness: Keep a diary of my foods. I am accountable.

Day 2: Water: Sip half my body weight in ounces throughout the day.

Day 3: Movement: Some exercise performed every day. Note it in my diary.

Day 4: Regular meals: Eat about the same time each day.

Day 5: Vegetables and Raw Living Foods: 50% of total weight of your food.

So here is the list of foods you can eat in abundance!

Eat all you want but at least 50% of total weight of the meal		*none of these are considered vegetables unless raw*
artichoke	jicama	beet
arugula	kale	carrot *(cooked)*
asparagus	kelp	corn
bamboo shoots	leek	daikon *(cooked)*
beet greens	lettuce *(all varieties)*	parsnip
bok choy	mushroom *(all varieties)*	peas *(cooked)*
broccoli	mustard greens	potato
Brussels sprouts	okra	pumpkin
cucumber	onion	rutabaga
cabbage	parsley	squash winter
cactus nopales	peas & pea pods *(raw)*	sweet potato
carrot *(raw)*	peppers *(all varieties)*	turnip
caulifower	radicchio	yam
celery	radish	yucca
cilantro	spinach	
collard greens	sprouts *(all varieties)*	
daikon *(raw)*	squash summer	
eggplant	Swiss chard	
endive	tomato	
fennel	turnip greens	
garlic	water chestnut	
ginger	watercress	
green beans	zucchini	

Day 6
Fruit

Let's set the record straight about a food which has been considered a healthy food for a very long time: FRUIT!

In Nature, the fruit is the part of the plant which carries the seed. It is often bright in color, sweet in taste, aromatic in odor and attractive to animals. Nature does this so that animals will eat the fruit, digest it, and hopefully wander far enough afield where they finally poop it out in a place where the seed can produce a new plant far from its parent. The poop is full of special fertilizer to nurture the future seedling and get it going. (But please watch your step!)

For the purposes of this book, we will refer to a fruit a plant food which carries the plant's seed and which is SWEET. Although tomatoes, cucumbers, peppers, beans and squash are all actually fruits, we will refer to them as vegetables because they are low in sugar.

That which we call fruit, and which we find in our grocery stores today, is really not so natural. These types of fruit were not originally found in Nature. Are you raising your eyebrows in disbelief? It is true; this fruit as found in the grocery store was never created by Nature, at least not in its current form. It's been hybridized, genetically manipulated and bred repeatedly by human scientists to create something very different from its prehistoric ancestors.

Because we humans have a sweet tooth and are driven by our taste buds, we have manipulated the plants' genes to create fruit which is large, juicy and full of sugar. In fact, the sugar in some of these fruits is equal to what we would find in junk food! You heard correctly. A banana and an orange each has 17 grams of sugar and a medium sized apple has 19 grams. This is significant when you consider that a McDonald's chocolate chip cookie has only 15 grams! Just when you thought you were doing the right thing for your body all these years by eating fruit instead of that cookie you really wanted!

Now take this one step farther. These unnatural, genetically manipulated fruits are harvested and condensed into foods which are even less natural than the already unnatural fruit. Fruit juices are made from them by squeezing the concentrated liquid from them. Some fruit juice companies even add more sugar and artificial color to this juice to make it taste sweeter and look prettier. What is left behind and discarded is the very important fiber within which Nature packaged the fruit!

Think about how much fruit it takes to make just one glass of juice. Did you know it takes three to five pieces of fruit to make a single glass of juice? You might as well trade that in for a whole handful of chocolate chip cookies! (Do you like chocolate chip cookies as much as I do?) Actually, you could even trade it in for a Coke™ because a glass of OJ has just as many grams of sugar! That's right: one 8 ounce cup of OJ and one 8 ounce cup of Coke each have 26 grams of sugar. That is more than 6 teaspoons of sugar! Wow! Could you have enough room in your tummy for three to five pieces of fruit with the rest your meal if they were in whole food form? There wouldn't be much room left for eggs, bacon and pancakes if that were the case.

While we are on the subject, it is fair to mention that even vegetable juice should be prepared and consumed cautiously. Most people consider freshly made vegetable juice a very nutritious health food and it certainly is loaded with minerals and vitamins. If you prepare your own juice at home you want to make sure it is made from mostly green vegetables and NOT just carrots and apples and beets. Carrot/apple/beet juices taste good because they are naturally sweet. Be aware that this so-called healthy vegetable juice can affect sugar levels as much as fruit juice. If you make your own juice at home, be sure it is no more than 50% carrot/apple/beet and the other 50% made from green vegetables like celery, cucumber, kale, collard greens, lettuce, green beans and anything else green you can find.

Sugars of all types can be harmful to people who already have elevated blood sugar levels. If you know your fasting glucose is above 99 mg/dL then you should really avoid fruit and fruit juice altogether. If your waist line is greater than 40 inches for a man and 35 inches for the woman, you are possibly already experiencing insulin resistance even if it is not showing up in your lab tests yet. In either case, you should not treat fruit or fruit juice as a health food and it should only be consumed occasionally.

Nature designed the juice of vegetables and fruit to be eaten with the fiber. Nature gave us the fruit in a whole package for a reason! Have you ever seen chimpanzees sipping a glass of OJ to start their days? How about gorillas blending up a banana fruit smoothie? It's just not what Nature intended. The fiber found in the whole fruit serves an important purpose: to slow the absorption of the fruit sugars into the system.

Fizzy Ferments

You are probably quite aware of what happens when you eat too much fruit. You get "the squirts" or "the runs" as we used to call it as kids! (Some words are just graphic enough to tell the whole story.) If too much fruit sugar, or fructose as it is called, is eaten, it passes into the intestines where bacteria break it down and it can cause bloating, gas, and loose stools. The naturally occurring yeast organisms which live in your gut may also act on simple sugars like glucose or fructose and convert them to ethanol and carbon dioxide. Do you know what other types of drink also contains those two ingredients? How do you make a bubbly beverage? Add in fruit or grain, yeast, and time… and you have the beginning of champagne or moonshine or any other alcoholic beverage!

In fact, people who have tendencies to yeast (candida) infections and fungal infections should avoid fruit, refined carbohydrates and sugar products as it serves only to feed these little yeasty guys and helps them to multiply. Cut off the yeast's food supply and you reduce their population, which means you alleviate your symptoms. Also, it is important to note that people who are highly attracted to sugar and fruit are actually making ethanol or alcohol in their guts. As sugar is ingested into their systems, it mixes with the yeasts in their gut which in turn converts the sugar into alcohol.

Many people who have never had an addiction to drugs or alcohol have a strong addiction to chocolate or sugar. That is right! SUGAR-aholics can be chemically making alcohol in their gut! Small wonder it is such a strong addiction, and this is especially important to keep in mind if alcohol addiction runs in the family. Decreasing sugar intake will decrease the internal production of alcohol which, in turn, will decrease the chances for relapses or addictions.

Another form of fruit to approach carefully is dehydrated fruit. Dehydrating foods is a method of preservation used for thousands of years by our ancestors. It is a very effective way to keep food from spoiling without refrigeration. However, these foods are very concentrated. Like juice without the fiber, dehydrated fruits are not what Nature intended. Without their water, they are smaller and you are able to eat more than what you would be able to eat fresh. And it is important to note that when a food is dehydrated it takes water from your body in order to rehydrate itself.

The high concentration of sugar does not make food like dates, prunes, raisins, craisins or any other dried fruit a good choice, especially for diabetics or those trying to lose weight. It is a double whammy negative for someone who has higher amounts of yeast in his or her digestive tract. Again, the high sugar feeds the yeast and the byproduct is fermentation and alcohol. Dehydrated fruits are only acceptable if used moderately and only then if first rehydrated in water overnight before eating. They can also be used as sweetener or flavoring when cooked with foods like grains. A small handful of raisins or dehydrated prunes added to whole grain cereal or oatmeal while it is cooking can provide some needed flavor.

Fruit Thieves! Stolen at the Peak of Perfection!

But there are qualities of fruit which are very healthful. When fruit is allowed to ripen to maturity on the vine, it is loaded with vitamins, bioflavonoids, antioxidants and other phytochemicals. These are the beneficial nutrients which give fruit the health qualities you have heard about. I am most impressed with the chemicals called bioflavonoids. I feel one day they will be in the forefront of preventive medicine of the future.

Phytochemicals are what gives fruit its beautiful color. These pigments are made by the plant in response to the harsh rays of the sun which shine on it during the day. The pigments protect the plant from the sun as well as serve as a natural pesticide and protection against microorganism invaders. When you eat these powerful chemicals, they have a protective effect on you as they did on the plant. You might have heard of some of them: resveratrol, OPCs (Oligomeric proanthocyanidins), pycnogenol, quercetin, and EGCG (epigallocatechin gallate) all of which are making big news. They provide protection against oxidation and organ damage and they are also being studied for their powerful anti-aging properties.

The grocery store is not the best source from which to purchase fruit. Most fruit in the grocery store has been picked green instead of when it is mature and ripe. This is especially with fruit shipped from other countries. Have you seen the anemic "salmon colored" strawberries available in the dead of winter? Don't eat them, it is not their season. They were picked green and forced to grow by means of multiple chemicals prior to shipping. Have you seen the green bananas that eventually turn yellow over the weeks while sitting in piles at the grocery store? These fruits were not allowed to grow to maturity on the tree and picked at their peak. It is at maturation that the nutritional qualities of all fruit are also at their peak, providing minerals, antioxidants and don't forget biophotons.

I remember being a young boy and admiring the maturing cherries on the cherry tree in our backyard every summer. As children, we waited and watched day by day, excited to see the little cherries slowly plumping up and changing from green to yellow to pink to red. My sister and I counted the days when we could climb the tree so we could pluck the biggest, ripest, juiciest cherry of the bunch. I couldn't wait to pop it in my mouth and bite down on its sweet juicy crimson flesh. Well, little did I realize that my prized cherries were also being admired from afar by the local crows, robins, starlings, and blackbirds. They were lining up in the trees all around waiting like crazed shoppers in their tents outside their favorite store on Black Friday.

Sure enough, just like the crazed shoppers, the day the fruit was ripe and ready to eat, hordes of them came out of nowhere in a mad chaos of wings and feathers and beaks. I stood there helplessly, ready to cry, able to do nothing to save my preciously nurtured fruits as these varmints swooped in mercilessly and stole my delicious cherries at their peak of perfection. I was no match for these witty creatures and they cleaned out the entire tree in the matter of hours! Drat! Those creatures knew exactly when that fruit was at its sweetest and ready to burst with living activated nutrition and sun's energy. Nature knows best.

Live Under Your Own Fig Tree

In order to get fruit which is high in nutrition and antioxidants, choose to buy from farmer's markets and stores which stock locally grown produce. This fruit is most likely to have been picked at the peak of its perfection, as Nature intended. Also, choose to *eat fruit that is in season from your local area.* For example, don't eat strawberries or melons or any other fruit in the middle of winter if you live in a climate in which they can't be grown at that time of year. Besides, haven't you noticed that how anemic, hard and pithy, and totally lacking in flavor and aroma they are if they aren't fresh in the season? The same goes for all produce; it is best to eat the foods that are in season in your area.

Therefore, choose to only eat tropical fruit if you are living in the tropics. Live under your own fig tree as stated, "Every man under his vine and under his fig tree".[1] Besides, tropical fruit is some of the most sugary fruit of all. In general, the sweetest fruits will be found in the parts of the world which receive the most sunlight and the more tart fruits, such as apples and berries, will be found in cooler climates. Eating sweet fruits can be like eating candy, so if you are in the tropics and enjoying this fruit, make it only a couple pieces a day; a little goes a long way!

Choose fruit which still resembles its ancestors found growing wild in Nature. Nature originally made fruit rich in color, smaller in size, and lower in sugar. Berries of all types, plums, cherries, small purple grapes, and other fruits which are rich in color and flavor and lower in sugar are great choices. These are the fruits that science shows to be rich in the phytochemicals that slow the aging process and protect us from harmful chemicals in the environment.

Frozen and canned fruits, jams and preserves, as long as no extra sugar is added, are generally ok. The nice thing about some canned or frozen foods is that they are not picked before they're ripe. These are fruits which are picked at the peak of their maturity and tend to be rich in nutrients. But once again, remember that the amount you consume is what matters. You do not want to eat more than one serving of fruit at a time; this is approximately the equivalent of one cup. Fruit juice, as mentioned earlier, should be avoided because of its high concentration of sugar. Tomato juice, however, if stored in a glass container, can be a healthy source of antioxidants and it is low in carbohydrates.

A good time to eat fruit is as a snack between meals because it doesn't mix well with other foods; we will discuss that in more detail on day 11 in the section on food combinations. Also, fruit can be a good option for those who need something light with which to start the day. It is not adequate for a complete breakfast but some people may choose to have a little fruit 30 minutes to an hour before breakfast to get their digestive systems stimulated after the night's rest. Do not eat fruit within 30 minutes of a meal. Fruit makes a nice energy booster and is a light snack on the stomach before working out. Allow 20-30 minutes after eating fruit before you do any exercise.

[1] 1 Kings 4:25, Micah 4:4.

START TODAY:

- From here on, choose fruit that is in the most natural state possible. Choose fruit that is grown in your area and in season. Some fruits like apples which are able to be picked ripe and kept in cold storage throughout the winter are still be considered to be in season.

- Limit your consumption to no more than one serving of fruit, which is about a cup. Eating fruit is optional; you may choose to omit it altogether. It can be eaten a couple times per day and is great way to start the day, as a snack between meals, or before workouts. Make sure that it is not eaten with your meal.

- Eliminate all fruit juices or anything made with processed fruit, including fruit desserts, jams, jellies, fruit sauces or canned fruits with added sweetener. If they are made without additives then they are allowed.

Summary: This is what I'm doing up to this point, each day adds onto the next

Day 1: **Food awareness:** Keep a diary of my foods. I am accountable.

Day 2: **Water:** Sip half my body weight in ounces throughout the day.

Day 3: **Movement:** Some exercise performed every day. Note it in my diary.

Day 4: **Regular meals:** Eat about the same time each day.

Day 5: **Vegetables and Raw Living Foods:** 50% of total weight of your food.

Day 6: **Fruit:** Up to 2 servings of locally grown fruit daily (no fruit juice).

List of healthy fruit choices as an optional snack between meals:

Consider a serving to be approximately 1 cup of fresh fruit or ¼ cup for dried fruit

Apples	Grapes	Peaches
Apricots	Grapefruit	Persimmons
Bananas	Guava	Pineapple
Blackberries	Honeydew	Plums
Blueberries	Kiwis	Pomegranates
Boysenberries	Lemons	Prunes
Cantaloupe	Limes	Raisins
Cherries	Mangoes	Raspberries
Cranberries	Nectarines	Rhubarb
Dates	Oranges	Strawberries
Figs	Papaya	Tangerines
Gooseberries	Pears	Watermelon

Day 7
Carbohydrates, Starches, & Sugars

C ongratulations! You made it to the end of the first week! While we are on the topic of fruits and sugar, let's transition to a favorite food category for many of us: CARBS! Yes, indeed! They fit right in there with some of the greatest taste bud ticklers of all! Mmmm... fresh breads, Italian pastas, potato chips, pastries, cookies, donuts, and let's not forget about chocolate!!

As nummy as these foods are, if they are eaten more than occasionally, they can turn into a rolling ball of health problems. As we know, carbohydrates are starches which break down into sugar in the body. How much turns to sugar and how quickly it does depends on the type of starchy food eaten. Not all carbohydrates are created equal. In general, the more processed or refined the carbohydrate food is, the less beneficial and more harmful it is. Nature has already provided starches or carbohydrates in the forms which are most beneficial for the animals and for us. Humans do not need to change these perfect foods by processing and refining them. We only do this to make it more appealing to our palates.

For example, white rice is nothing more than brown rice with the outer husk polished off. This husk is the source of multiple nutrients, so when it is removed what is left behind is the soft inner white starchy grain of rice which is absorbed in the body much more rapidly without its harder brown fiber shell. The same is true for wheat. The whole wheat bread many of us buy in the store is really just white wheat flour bread with a dash of brown whole wheat flour added to give it a whole wheat appearance. True whole wheat sprouted bread is actually very dense, heavy, fibrous, and most people have to acquire a taste for it since it doesn't feel soft and squishy in the mouth.

In the United States particularly, we have grown accustomed to eating an abundance of food made from processed wheat: breads, pastries, pastas, rolls and buns, pizza dough, macaroni, cold cereal etc. Look at your personal food diary up to this point. Is there even one day that a wheat product wasn't eaten? If you are like the majority of my patients and the majority of Americans the answer is probably no. What does this mean for you?

Whole wheat is a natural whole grain and in its natural state it is a healthy grain like many others. What causes it to become undesirable is processing it in order to improve its taste. We then not only eat it processed, but we eat a WHOLE LOT OF IT in this processed form. Western countries eat more processed wheat than any other grain. Processing, remember, strips the food of it original nutrients and makes it a refined carbohydrate, which is absorbed more like white sugar in the body. And remember from yesterday, this fast carbohydrate absorption causes excess insulin to be released from the pancreas which is trying to push the high sugar into the cells. When insulin is released, it sends a message to the cells of the body: STORE FAT and DO NOT BURN FAT!

Insulin is the survival hormone. If you are overweight or if you have always struggled with your weight, you have actually been endowed with a strong adaptive mechanism that served your ancestors well. Your ancestors would have been more likely to survive famine because their insulin response to food was stronger than that of those who perished. Their bodies would take the excess energy from the limited amount of food they ate and store it as fat for the days during which there was no food. These days however, you are no longer in survival mode, but your genes still are! So when the cells perceive an increase of sugar in the blood stream, insulin says, "Store that, I may get hungry one day when there is no food!" Therefore, too many carbohydrate foods are not good for people wanting to lose weight because insulin will tell the body to store this excess as fat.

When you eat starchy or sugary foods regularly, insulin is also secreted regularly. The pancreas not only wears out from the constant production of insulin, but the body's cells become insensitive to insulin because it is at such high levels all the time. The body adjusts to this high amount of insulin and needs more and more of it to do the same job of lowering the blood sugar. This condition is called insulin resistance. The insulin is no longer able to push the sugar into the cells and the blood sugars continue to escalate. Diabetes is now right around the corner.

Variety is the Spice of Life

Eating grains such as wheat on a daily basis can cause problems for those who have food allergies. Although grains are mostly carbohydrates, they also contain proteins which can trigger allergies in people with immune dysfunctions. This is especially the case if they consume the same allergic foods day after day. If someone is experiencing seasonal allergies, asthma, skin rashes, intestinal irritability, constipation, or persistent colds and infections, it is quite possible that their immune system is reacting to the proteins found in some of their foods.

The culprits of these immune dysfunctions are the main proteins in wheat called gluten and gliadin. They are large proteins which, if not properly digested, can find their way into the bloodstream and cause an immune response. By simply reducing the amount of wheat you eat and substituting a wider variety of other types of carbohydrates, you can change how your body reacts to wheat-based foods. In fact, some people who once thought they were wheat-intolerant were actually just "wheated out." They ate too much wheat for too long and once they took a break from it for a while, were able to eat it again a couple times a week. As a clinician, I also recommend my patients who show symptoms potentially associated with food allergies to have an ELISA IgG food allergy test. See Sources.

In reality, there are very few carbohydrate foods which follow Nature's plan. For example, whole bran muffins are not a natural food. Neither is whole grain pasta, or ground corn tortillas, or your shredded wheat cereal or even that healthy whole grain sprouted grain bread! Why do you think? Well, have you seen many plant bushes that are producing tortilla chips or tortellinis ready to be picked and eaten? Even though these seem like healthful starches, they are, in reality, not considered to be food as prepared by Nature.

The entire concept of this book is to look to Nature for our answers to health. With this understanding, unless it is 100% prepared by Nature in a perfect package and ready to eat, it really is not natural. However, it is important for us to have enough variety so that we are able to have both enjoyment of our food and good health. The table of carbohydrates at the end of this chapter does recommend some carbohydrate foods which are not entirely natural, and some minimally processed carbohydrates have been included in order to provide some variety to your meals.

But remember, this program is not about always being a saint or a good girl or good boy. This is about getting into a good routine so that when you drift away from Nature's foods, such as when you're on vacation or are at a friend's house or are going out to eat a special meal, you can return to your everyday healthy lifestyle the next day. Nature's Diet is not something you do for a period of time to lose weight and then return back to your old ways. To bring lasting changes to your health, you will need to make lasting changes to the foods you eat. *This is not a diet fad, this is a lifestyle. This is forever*!

One category of carbohydrates which are particularly helpful in balancing health is the bean and legume family. These are classified as carbohydrates but they have enough protein and fiber that they are a slow burning carbohydrate and make excellent food for people with high blood sugars, or those trying to lose weight. Somebody had it right with that old ditty, "beans, beans the magical fruit!"

There are many types. Try them all, especially pintos, black, red, black-eyed peas, mung beans, and my favorites: brown lentils, red lentils, and green and yellow split peas. For those who have trouble digesting beans, lentils and split peas cause little or no digestive distress if prepared properly. By the way, green beans and snow peas are considered vegetables while dried beans and cooked green peas are considered to be starchy carbohydrates.

Fight of the Phytates

It is recommended that you have a variety of the carbohydrates listed at the end of the chapter. The more types you eat, the better your chances of receiving a wide variety of vitamins and minerals. This is especially important with grains. Instead of eating the same grains all the time, choose new grains which are not regularly in your diet. The greater variety of foods you eat, the less likely your body will respond with an immune response such as food allergies. Therefore try new grains like millet, quinoa (pronounce keen-wa), brown rice, red rice, wild rice, barley, amaranth, and any other grain that looks different and fun and new. Try it! Be brave!

Something to bear in mind is that the eating of grain-type foods is a relatively recent development in the history of the human race. Growing and eating grains has only developed within the last several thousand years.[1] Before this there was no farming; our ancestors fed themselves by hunting and gathering plants. Grains became a part of our diet later on as people began to grow food rather than gather it. This might explain another reason many people are allergic or sensitive to grains: our digestive and immune systems still haven't adapted to them. It might also explain why diabetes is so prevalent; the human body has not adapted to the high amount of carbohydrates provided by grains and our sugar-rich diets.

Interestingly, grains naturally contain chemicals called phytates. These substances are Nature's protective chemicals, found within the seed and which protect it from decay while it is waiting to germinate. If the phytates are not neutralized before the grain is ingested, they can bind the minerals calcium, magnesium, iron, and zinc and contribute to mineral deficiencies in your body. Phytates are neutralized by soaking, sprouting, or cooking the grains. Their effect is a greater concern for those who eat only grain, and most especially for children and the elderly in developing countries.

Instead of grains, root vegetables and members of the squash family are the carbohydrates of choice for those with sensitive stomachs and digestive complaints. Select the potato varieties which are smaller in size because they tend to concentrate more nutrients and are less starchy. The nutrients are most dense in the outermost half inch of the potato, just beneath the skin. The large roasting or baking potatoes are not the most desirable because they have a much higher ratio of starches to minerals. Choose baby red, yellow, purple, or blue potatoes. Yes, blue potatoes straight from Farmer Smurf! Amaze your friends and throw a rainbow potato party! Also, choose sweet potatoes and yams for a change for your taste buds and add a healthy boost to your much needed beta-carotene levels. Carrots, parsnips, beets, rutabagas and turnips are all excellent starches when cooked. Winter and summer squashes are rich in vitamins, especially the carotenes. I have found these to be the most gentle starches for healing an inflamed and irritable gut.

Don't Be a Hater

Remember that "carbs", as they are so-called by the "sugar haters" out there, are not all bad. Carbohydrates turn into glucose, which is the main fuel your body uses for energy and is essential for proper brain functioning. The problem with carbs occurs when you consume more than your body can burn. Carbohydrates also have another, more recently discovered, purpose.

Science has discovered that some sugars have medicinal properties and very important roles in immune system functions. Eight separate essential sugars, or glyconutrients, have been discovered as needed by the body. They are fucose, galactose, glucose, mannose, n-acetylgalactosamine, n-acetylglucosamine, n-acetylneuraminic acid and xylose. Of these eight essentials, only glucose and galactose are found in the majority of our diets. These eight complete sugars would be found in Nature's Diet abundant with organic vegetables and fruits, homegrown in fertile soil and allowed to ripen to maturity. They are also what give plants like aloe vera, noni fruit, and medicinal mushrooms their powerful healing properties.

These essential sugars are utilized on the surface membranes of your cells and are needed so your cells can talk to one another. Think of your cells like teenagers that need to stay connected with their friends via text messages and rollover minutes. The benefit to you is that as long as these teens don't run out of "minutes" (these essential simple sugars) they can let the rest of their friends know how they are doing. They can tell the other cells if they have excesses or deficiencies of nutrients, if they are overloaded with toxins or poisons, if they have been taken over by a virus or parasite, or if the cells have become cancerous. If this communication is happening effectively, the cells can alert the immune system troops so they can haul off a sick or infected cell. These essential sugars, or glyconutrients, display powerful immune system support against auto-immune illnesses and conditions like cancer, AIDS, and any other forms of immune system suppression.

Your Gut Instinct

Now back to your starches. So how much is too much? Very good question. Again, this should be simple, nothing too exacting; that is not so necessary. If you make healthy carbohydrate choices and you combine them properly with other foods, they will not have a strong sugar releasing effect. They will be healthful and not damaging; that information comes up shortly.

If the goal is to consume about half the weight of our food in vegetables, the average person would want about ¼ of the weight of their meal to be carbohydrates. This would be the equivalent of about 25-35 grams of complex carbohydrate per meal. (see table) But, because we are all biochemically unique, this is also going to depend on how well you process carbohydrates. Let's ask your own gut instinct.

1) Are you someone who can go a long time without eating?
2) Are you someone who feels satisfied with a light meal?
3) Are you someone who has a sluggish or weak digestion?

If you answered yes to more than one of these questions, then it is likely your genes are telling you that your body is made for foods which are lighter and easier to digest. This means you would do better with foods from plants or a vegetarian-inclined diet. If this is the case, you should follow what your body is telling you. Because carbohydrates and plant foods are easier to digest than protein and fat foods, you should increase the proportion of starches to about 1 ½ servings of a carbohydrate in the table below or about 40-50 grams per meal. In other words, instead of one cup of cooked brown rice, your body needs more like 1 ½ cups of cooked brown rice at that meal.

On the other hand if you answered no to these questions; if you find yourself constantly hungry, if you have a strong digestion, or if you don't feel satisfied with simple light vegetarian meals then you are likely to be someone who doesn't need as much starch per meal. You will actually be someone that does better with meat or the protein type which we'll discuss next. In your case, eat less than the recommended ¼ plate of carbohydrates. Your range would be somewhere between 10-20 grams of carbohydrates per meal. For example, instead of one cup of cooked potato as an average serving, you would eat ½ cup cooked potato per meal.

If you don't answer with strong responses in either category above then you can assume your carbohydrate amount is in the average range and 1/4 plate of carbohydrates would be appropriate for you.

If you want to mix and match more than one carbohydrate at a meal simply do not exceed one serving of the combined starches. For example, if you wish to have rice and beans both of which are listed as one cup per serving, simply enjoy ½ cup of cooked rice and ½ cup of cooked beans to equal one total serving at that meal. If, like Forrest Gump, you wish to have peas and carrots, combine ½ cup of cooked peas and ½ cup of cooked carrots to equal one complete serving.

START TODAY:

- Add carbohydrates to your meals as long as they are balanced with your generous servings of vegetables at the same meal. The vegetables will be about ½ the weight of your total meal and the carbohydrate portion will be about ¼ of the weight of your total meal

- If you are more of a vegetarian type (determined above), eat 1 ½ servings below

- If you are more of a protein type (determined above), reduce the starch from the average portion to about ½ the average serving below.

- Sensitive folks should avoid wheat and other grains and instead choose carbohydrates from roots, squashes, peas and legumes.

[1]It is estimated that humans began cultivating food for agricultural purposes between 3,000 and 10,000 years ago at different times for different parts of the world.

Carbohydrate Options: *The amounts listed are based on a COOKED serving size and are considered to be average serving sizes. Choose one serving per meal which is about 25–35 grams carbohydrates*

GRAINS *1 cup cooked*	ROOTS *Amounts listed*	SQUASH *1 ½ cups*	BEANS, PEAS *1 cup cooked*	PROCESSED GRAINS= *25-35 g/serving*
amaranth	beet *3c*	all winter squash	adzuki beans	corn tortilla *(3 small)*
barley	carrots *2c*	acorn squash	black beans	whole grain sprouted breads *(2 slices)*
brown rice	daikon radish *2c*	banana squash	black-eyed peas	tortilla chips *1 oz (20 chips)*
buckwheat	Jerusalem artichoke *1c*	butternut squash	fava beans	brown rice cakes *(4 small)*
corn kernels	parsnip *2c*	delicata squash	garbanzo beans	shredded wheat cereal *(3/4 cup)*
corn grits	potato *1c (any type)*	hubbard squash	green peas	whole grain pasta *(3/4 cup)*
kamut	rutabaga *2c*	pumpkin	great northern beans	whole grain corn bread *(1 piece)*
millet	sweet potato *1c*	spaghetti squash	kidney beans	rice pasta *(3/4 cup)*
oat meal	turnip *3c*	sweet meat squash	lentils	corn pasta *(3/4 cup)*
quinoa	yam *1c*		lima beans	rye crisp crackers *(8)*
red rice	yucca *1c*		mung beans	rice crackers *(1½ oz)*
rye			navy beans	sprouted grain bagel *(½)*
spelt			pinto beans	sprouted grain pita *(1 large)*
triticale			red beans	flax seed crackers *(1½ oz)*
wheat			soy beans	
wild rice			split peas	
			tofu	
			white beans	

EXTRAS:

apple sauce *1c*

rice milk/soy milk *8oz* often contain 25-35 grams carbohydrate

coconut yogurt *6oz.*
soy yogurt *6oz*

Summary: This is what I'm doing up to this point, each day adds onto the next

Day 1: **Food awareness:** Keep a diary of my foods. I am accountable.

Day 2: **Water:** Sip half my body weight in ounces throughout the day.

Day 3: **Movement:** Some exercise performed every day. Note it in my diary.

Day 4: **Regular meals:** Eat about the same time each day.

Day 5: **Vegetables and Raw Living Foods:** 50% of total weight of your food.

Day 6: **Fruit:** Up to 2 servings of locally grown fruit daily (no fruit juice).

Day 7: **Carbohydrates:** One serving per meal combined with vegetables.

Day 8
Protein

How is it coming along? Starting to get the hang of this yet? Now onto one of the most controversial subjects of all: PROTEIN!

"To eat meat or not to eat meat?" That is the question

Vegetarianism, Macrobiotics, Zone, Blood Type, Atkins, Pritikin, South Beach, etc, etc, etc... the list can be exhausting, confusing, and painstaking....and without achieving results, downright depressing. It seems the authors have either a "fascinating fetish for flesh" or complete disgust for carnivorism, calling for a national moratorium on the ingestion of "bacteria-infested maggot food!" As you can see, there are widely disparate and often passionate opinions on the subject.

Those who claim vegetarianism is the only way to eat say that we should imitate the apes and chimps, who are vegan vegetarians. Those that claim carnivorism is more appropriate for humans argue that the Inuit Eskimos are in excellent health surviving mostly on fish and meat. What does Nature say? Remember, Nature provides every answer to our questions. All we have to do is open our eyes, ears, and mind, and pay attention to the answers all around us.

We humans are as diverse chemically as we are physically. Our chemical diversity means there are different needs for different people which in turn means there is no single best diet for all people. Hence, what has worked for one person may or may not work for someone else. No wonder there are so many diets, and they all work, for SOME people!!! Each person's physiological needs differ widely depending on genetic make-up, environmental factors, caloric demands from physical activity, and many other factors.

Protein is considered the most important macromolecule in the body as it was named after the Greek root meaning "in the lead" or "first in rank" which tells us just how important these compounds are. Protein makes up about one half of the dry weight of your body which means it is second only to water in total content. When the protein in your food is digested it breaks down into 22 simple amino acids, including the 8 essential amino acids which the body cannot produce by itself. Obviously, this means that if you aren't eating quality protein, you will not be getting these essential nutrients. Once digested, these amino acids then re-combine to make biological proteins which are utilized to form the structure of every single cell in your body from your heart to your skin to your bones to your eyeballs!

Bones aren't simply calcium; if they were you'd be as brittle as chalk and break like a twig! About 50% of the composition of your bones is minerals and the other 50% is water, protein and fat. A protein called collagen is the substance which gives your skin a soft, youthful appearance. When collagen breaks down, the results are those dreaded wrinkles. Even the hair on your head and the nails on your hands and feet are made from a protein called keratin. Hair and nails are considered to be non-essential protein structures. If your body isn't getting enough protein from your diet or if it requires more protein during times of starvation or times of illness, the hair will fall and the nails will grow weak or ridged. Your body will actually sacrifice hair and nails so that it has enough protein for more essential functions. Do you know anyone with falling hair or weak brittle nails?

Amino acids are essential to make hormones and neurotransmitters like insulin from the pancreas, thyroxine from the thyroid, adrenaline from the adrenals and serotonin from the brain, among others. Amino acids combine to make immunoglobulins and antibodies which are the arsenal your immune system uses to fight off invaders. Hemoglobin is the main protein in the red blood cells which combines with iron to supply oxygen to the cells.

All the enzymes in your body, from those which accelerate chemical reactions to those which digest food, are all proteins made from amino acids. Every one of these hundreds of thousands of proteins which in turn are composed of hundreds of thousands of amino acids are constructed continuously by the magical code inside each of 100 trillion cells in your body: DNA and RNA. Do you see how vitally important it is that your body receives all the necessary amino acid building blocks?

Monkey Business

To gain an insight of the proper balance of foods needed by a human it is important for us to look towards Nature. Here we can observe the natural habits of our closest relatives who have not been indoctrinated into the modern habits of Western living. The food intake of wild primates around the world has been observed and some of the findings are described in this encyclopedia excerpt: [1]

> The primate order includes a handful of species that live entirely on meat (carnivores) and also a few that are strict vegetarians (herbivores), but it is composed chiefly of animals that have varied diets (omnivores). The carnivorous primates are the four species of tarsiers, which live in Southeast Asia. Using their long back legs, these pocket-sized nocturnal hunters leap on their prey, pinning it down with their hands and then killing it with their needle-sharp teeth. Tarsiers primarily eat insects but will also eat lizards, bats, and snakes... This opportunistic approach to feeding is seen in the majority of monkeys and also in chimpanzees. Several species of monkeys, and chimpanzees, but not the other apes, have been known to attack and eat other monkeys. Baboons, the most adept hunters on the ground, often eat meat and sometimes manage to kill small antelope.

Most apes and monkeys eat a range of plant-based foods, but a few specialize in eating leaves. South American howler monkeys and African colobus monkeys eat the leaves of many different trees, but the proboscis monkey on the island of Borneo is more selective, surviving largely on the leaves of mangroves. These leaf-eating monkeys have modified digestive systems, similar to cows, which enable them to break down food that few other monkeys can digest. Other apes and monkeys eat mostly fruit, while some marmosets and lemurs depend on tree gum and sap.[1]

AMAZING! Amazing to see how diverse the food demands can be in an animal family so closely related to us humans. The animal's environmental conditions, the physical demands placed on their bodies, and the foods which are readily available, are the primary factors in their food choices and how they have adapted.

This holds true for humans, too. Observing the traditional diets of societies isolated from Western civilization and comparing it with the diets of our biological cousins the primates, has given us insightful clues to proper living as Nature intended. Modern man's food supply, like that of the primates, can range from mostly vegetarian to carnivorous to omnivorous. This is dependent on genetic background, geographical location, ambient temperature, and physical demands.

So, are humans built more like the meat-eating variety or more like the vegetarian variety? This is a tough question to answer with certainty but more clues can be seen if we pay closer attention to Nature. Nature designed the meat eaters with sharp pointy teeth for tearing flesh, claws for ripping the skin, and a shorter digestive tract that was high in acidity for digesting meat and killing bacteria on the meat. Vegetarians on the other hand, think of cows for instance, do not have claws, or fangs, but rather flat broad teeth for masticating and chewing fibrous material. They also have longer digestive systems including multiple stomachs that will break down the fibers into smaller and smaller molecules for digestion.

Humans are really a blend of both types. We have canine teeth which are our Dracula-like fangs for tearing! We also have our molars for grinding and mashing. We have a stomach that is rich in hydrochloric acid to break down meat and sizzle bacteria. We also have a pancreas that secretes enzymes to break down carbohydrates, fats, and proteins as well as a digestive tract that is 29 feet long and which is full of bacteria to break down carbohydrates and plant material. We have the best of both worlds! From this observation and comparing our digestive system to our closest relative the chimpanzees, we can assume that we are omnivorous. The specific amount of protein per person is dependent on the individual's genetic needs, his lifestyle, and his environment.

A Long Time Ago In a Galaxy Far, Far Away

In the 1930's, a dentist named Weston Price sought out the world's most traditional societies and performed one of the most famous epidemiological studies of all time. Price and his wife traveled more than 100,000 miles to study the health of isolated communities in Australia, Africa, South America, Polynesia, Europe, and northern Canada. He studied the oral health of those on native diets by counting cavities and examining tooth crowding and palate size. He compared the teeth of indigenous people sustained solely by their native diet with those who ate refined and processed food from the Western settlers living near the villages.

As one might expect, those isolated individuals eating Nature's foods that were highly mineralized and unprocessed had significantly better oral health than any of the people whose diet included refined foods. Within just one generation, the effect of those indigenous people eating the Westerner's diet was notable. The number of cavities per person living solely on traditional native foods was almost zero compared to rampant decay noted in those eating refined foods from Westerners. Moreover, after one generation, the indigenous people who ate processed foods began to show a tendency to having smaller palates resulting in over-crowded and crooked teeth. The people on native diets retained the wide palates, the sizes of their mouths remained the same and their teeth remained straight without overcrowding. Is there an association between the high levels of decay and braces seen in today's youth and their intake of junk food?

Dr. Price observed that northern natives, like the Inuit Eskimo who dieted predominantly on animal products, fared as well physically, if not better, than those who lived in warmer equatorial countries and dieted on a primarily plant-based diet. The environment in which the person lived provided the proper amount of macro and micronutrients ensuring good health and strong stature for a person living in that climate. After observing dozens of indigenous societies, Price concluded that vegetarianism was not the dietary answer for every human. Rather, he noted that those sustaining an omnivorous diet had better oral health than those who were solely vegetarian. More importantly though, he found that to maintain nutritional levels the foods were to be eaten in a whole and unprocessed natural form.

His observations proved to be a historical breakthrough for advances in human nutrition and the benefits of traditional foods. Using Price's study as a template of proper nutrition, one can infer that a single diet for all humans would not be appropriate because multiple factors determine the specific dietary needs for each individual. These again are determined by their genetic ancestry, the demands of their lifestyle in work and play, and the temperature of their climate. If you wish to read more about Price's work you should read his book, *Nutrition and Physical Degeneration*.

It is still debatable whether our early ancestors were primarily hunters of meat or scavengers of meat. It is likely that our ancient ancestors were not the fierce hunters we like to envision, with bulging muscles sporting loin cloths and toting clubs and spears. More than likely, we came in and cautiously ate the remains of the animals after a carnivore had already killed them for us. In the Middle Ages, meat was limited in supply and was an expensive commodity eaten mostly by royalty and the aristocracy. Today in the Western world, meat is widely available but it is still the most expensive food type due to the costs of raising livestock.

Vegans Falling from Trees

Through clinical experience and by having once been a vegan myself, I have developed my own opinions about the practice of strict veganism. A Vegan vegetarian is a person who eats only plant-based foods. No dairy products, eggs, fish, poultry, or any meat or animal products of any type are consumed. Many of my patients who ate only vegan foods for an extended period of time (years) began to show deficiency symptoms associated with diets deficient in certain nutrients. My personal observations led me to conclude that those people who consume even very small quantities of animal protein have better health than those who are solely strict vegan vegetarians.

It is a well known fact that strict vegans develop vitamin B12 deficiencies if they are to abstain from all animal products. A deficiency of vitamin B12 can result in pernicious anemia, which can affect the nervous system and even be fatal if untreated. Now think about this: would Nature intend for us to be strict vegans if we would become extinct as a species from a lack of B12? I'm going to guess a big "NO" on that one. Maybe if Nature intended for us to be vegans, it would have provided a plant from which we could harvest little B12 vitamins as its fruit?

As silly as it sounds to pick vitamins from trees, it is true that a vegan diet needs to be supplemented with a pharmaceutical vitamin or animal sourced supplement because it does not supply the essential nutrients found in animal products. Nature does not provide vegetarian sources of vitamin B12 in any great quantity or absorbable form. Isn't it then reasonable to rule out a strict vegan diet as an ideal day-to-day diet for humans? If it was the ideal diet, we would not get anemia nor run the risk of our species becoming extinct as a result of avoiding animal products.

Please understand though, that the vegan diet has a very important purpose and can be an incredibly healthful diet for some people for a period of time. I will purposely prescribe a vegan diet to some of my patients if their lab values are indicating need for a diet which is less concentrated. In particular, I will choose to put patient on a vegan diet if they show YANG qualities like being too hot, having a red face, and a big round belly. They will also tend to improve on a vegan diet if they have health conditions such as high cholesterol, high blood pressure, or high blood sugar. This is also helpful for individuals with inflammatory or auto-immune conditions. In these cases, a strict vegan diet would be prescribed for a period of time sometimes for a year or longer until the individual became more balanced. When their values have normalized I'll recommend transitioning to Nature's Diet before they begin to show any signs of B12 deficiency.

Different Strokes for Different Folks

Not all proteins are made the same. Animal proteins are valuable because they contain the full spectrum of amino acids found in one complete package. Vegetable proteins have to be combined with multiple types of plant foods to get the wide assortment of amino acids and to compensate for their lack of the amino acid lysine. All amino acids needed by the structure of the human body and its metabolic needs are found in one serving of animal protein. Since we don't assimilate 100% of the food we put in our mouth, it is fair to say that some of that protein will be thrown off as waste instead of being used to rebuild tissue.

Vegetable protein is also less efficient than animal protein. Breast milk is the most efficient and usable protein at about 82% Utilizable Amino Acids (UAA). It is particularly high in glutamine, proline, and the branched chained amino acids. That leaves only 18% to be excreted as waste or used for energy and the rest for biological maintenance. This makes breast milk the most efficient protein available and the reason why it is so important for a newborn baby's development into childhood. Too bad it isn't readily found in the milk aisle! Eggs are 48% utilized and protein powder whey or soy supplements are just 16% utilized! This means the remaining 84% of the whey or soy protein powders, mostly used by athletes and weight lifters, is actually putting stress on the kidneys to remove the nitrogen waste instead of building muscle.[2]

How much animal protein does the human being need to meet the requirements for its physiology? Again you have to look selectively at what your individual body is telling you. Start utilizing those Natural instincts we have forgotten about. Again ask the questions we asked with the carbohydrates.

1) Are you someone who is hungry all the time?
2) Are you someone who needs protein at the meal to feel satisfied?
3) Are you someone with a cast-iron stomach who can eat anything?

If you answered yes to more than one of these questions, then it's likely your genes are telling you your body has the built-in mechanisms to require more protein and fat in your meals. So you should heed the cues that Nature is giving you.

Which Type are You?

People with inherently stronger digestive systems and appetites will have a natural craving and desire for meat. Those who don't will say that they don't feel well when eating meat. These people should eat lighter meat proteins like breast of fowl and fish and eat it in smaller amounts at each of the three meals (even if it is a single bite). Even if you are someone who has no desire for meat, you will still want to include a small amount in your diet. Some cravings are helpful for directing our food choices; some are not so good. Cravings for vegetables, salad, or "a good steak" are often leading us to a valid nutritional need by the body while cravings for chocolate or other sweets are cravings with empty promises.

Again, if you are someone who is often hungry between meals, not satisfied with vegetarian meals and you have a stomach which can digest rocks, then you should gravitate toward protein and fat-dominant meals. You should choose about 4 ounces of meat, fish, or eggs per meal, emphasizing richer red meats like grass-fed beef, lamb, buffalo, and wild game. Chose oilier fishes like salmon, and dark portions of poultry like thighs, wings, and legs. Your body is craving higher energy foods for a reason! Listen to it!

If you answered "no" to the three questions above then you have a body type which does better with lighter or predominately vegetarian meals. In your case you should choose 2 ounces or less of meat, fish, or eggs per meal. You may find you feel better with proteins which are easier to digest, such as eggs, fish, poultry and lean meat like buffalo or venison. If a medium sized egg is about 1 ½ ounces, 2 eggs would be an average of 3 ounces. Again, you should not go completely vegan; you should still have some animal products in your diet.

If you are a vegetarian and having difficulty with the idea of eating meat and feeling a little sick to your stomach, then just start with baby steps. Start by having a little organic chicken broth, just an ounce or two, warmed with salt and seasoning. Most people, even strict vegans, have no problem with this. When you have built up a taste for animal protein with broths, move onto eggs and then fish and then whatever you are able to tolerate. Remember, it doesn't need to be more than a bite or two in the beginning.

You may not fall into either of these extreme categories. If you are a person who doesn't have a craving for large amounts of meat or if vegetarian meals are not quite satisfying enough for you then you are in the middle of the road somewhere between the extremes. You are considered to have a more balanced digestion and you will do well with about 3 ounces of meat, fish or eggs per meal. See the table at the end of the chapter for complete animal protein selections. (These protein amounts are based on total ounces of animal product of meat, fish, or egg whole food. The actual amount of protein per serving of animal product would be about 18 grams per serving per meal).

A note about beef: it is not the bad guy it has been painted to be in the media. First of all, meat in general is not the villain that it has been made out to be all these years. Our ancestors ate meat as they roamed the lands since the beginnings of human existence. Only in recent times has agriculture developed and mankind started eating grains and other starches as staples.[3] Red meat is just as natural as any other meat as long as it has been raised naturally like the wild game your ancestors consumed. Remember, at one time our distant ancestors only ate what they could catch or kill; they did not raise animals in barns and feed them artificial feed. Our ancestors ate wild deer, elk, buffalo and moose, all of which are excellent sources of protein. These animals eat the foods Nature provided for them: grass, roots, and bark. These are all very low in fats and can result in meat that is high in essential fatty acids.

You are what you eat! Animals are what they eat, too! Conventionally raised beef (this is the beef you eat in most restaurants and purchase from the store) are fed grain and corn and soy (and God forbid - other cattle). These high energy starches help to artificially fatten the animal so that it produces meat with thick fatty marbling and – Mmm! - tastes good to us when that fat hits the grill! We are animals who LOVE FAT!! This thick marbling tastes good to us but couldn't be farther from a healthful choice for our bodies (more on the fat in meats on Day 9). So if you eat red meat, make sure the beef is free-range organic or a grass-fed beef. Even better, if you know someone who hunts wild game, see if they will part with some; you are talking about the cleanest meat available. Please realize that animals are higher up the food chain than vegetables and can accumulate toxins in their fat so it is very important that at the very least, you buy meats as clean as possible for your family.

Raw Savages

Back to the meat. Is the suggested amount of animal protein: 2, 3, or 4 ounces per meal, raw or cooked weight? That depends on whether you eat it raw or cooked. In the world where Nature was king, there was only raw meat! What? Yes, yes, yes, I'm talking pure and utter blasphemy! What filth! How disgusting! What an outcry! Once again, let's calmly look at Nature's plan and ask, "What would Nature do?" Well, sorry to say it folks, but have you ever seen a pack of wolves sitting back and shooting the breeze while roasting their Angus steaks, sipping Jack Daniels and smoking Marlboros? Well, maybe they do, but we're not likely to ever see it. It is like that old question about whether or not a falling tree makes noise in the forest when no one is there to hear it.

So it brings us back to another very important question. If Nature intended for us to eat cooked meat, wouldn't She have provided it in that form? Man has been cooking food many thousands of years, though it's only a fraction of human existence. Man is the only animal species which deliberately utilizes fire for heat and cooking. So it is fair to say that food, including meat, has been consumed in both the cooked and the raw form by our ancestors. It is also fair to say that the cooking of meat is not necessary for life because thousands of animal species would have become extinct long before this if their meat required cooking.

Although it is not done by other animal species, cooking of the food by humans can actually work in our favor. Cooking helps to "denature" or "break-down" complex protein molecules. This is exactly what our digestive juices and enzymes are designed to do to the protein we eat. Therefore cooking "pre-digests" the food by breaking down the cell walls of plants and the cell membranes of animal protein and makes it more assimilable.[4,5]

Cooking, as does freezing, drying, sprouting, fermenting and other preservation methods, breaks down the cell walls and membranes of our foods, allowing simpler nutrients to be more easily absorbed. Pre-digestion through cooking means that less digestive strength from our body is needed to break down food. Cooking food actually helped in the distant past to insure the survival of the human species. Early humans who were weak, sick or had compromised digestion were more likely to survive by eating food that was cooked. Cooking denatured the protein and made it more easily digested and utilized by their already weakened bodies.

Cautiously Cooking

Although cooking can make food more easily digested, the amount of nutrition destroyed by cooking is one of the disadvantages. Studies have shown that heat destruction can considerably decrease the amino acids in the protein which are the building blocks for our body. High heat used for long period of time is significantly more damaging than low heat ("slow and low") or short cycles of "flash heating". Heat significantly decreases the content of lysine, cystine, arginine, glutamic acid, glutamine, and aspartic acid pools by up to 40%![6,7] Cooking food can also destroy the soluble iron by 50% and the heme iron by 62% compared to raw meat.[8] Heme iron found in animal protein is the most absorbable form of iron and is best taken for those who are anemic.

Raw meat would be an ideal source of nutrition if we were able to have it fresh from the animal and eat it like animals did in the wild. As eating live vegetables from living plants is beneficial because of the activated and energetic cellular nutrients they contain, so are the activated nutrients from raw animal cells. Activated enzymes in the raw animal tissue are transferred to our bodies for utilization when we eat them; these would be destroyed by the heat of cooking. Vitamins and minerals are preserved in their most absorbable and assimilable forms when they are not broken down by cooking.

The really negative effects of cooking meat may have more to do with the effect it has on the oxidation of cholesterol and amino acid by-products which are formed than it has with nutrient destruction. There have been multiple studies showing the effect of heat on meats, particularly on grilling, which creates chemical by-products (polycyclic aromatic hydrocarbons and heterocyclic amines (PAHs, HCAs) which are known to increase cancer risk.[9,10]

Research conducted by the National Cancer Institute Division of Cancer Epidemiology and Genetics found a link between individuals with stomach, colorectal, pancreatic and breast cancer to be associated with high intakes of well-done, fried, broiled or barbecued meats. *People who eat medium-well or well-done beef were more than three times as likely to suffer stomach cancer as those who ate rare or medium-rare beef.*[11] The longer the meat is exposed to the high heat the more of these dangerous chemicals are formed. For many years there have been scare tactics convincing us to eat less meat. Now there are indications that meat inherently isn't bad; rather, any negative effect from meat is more likely due to the quality of the meat (conventional versus free range organic) and how it is prepared (high heat versus low heat).

Ideally, Nature would have us eat the meat fresh from the animal immediately after it was killed. If that wasn't possible, we would have taken it home as dry storage and heat it over a fire to burn off any bacterial decay. In a nutshell, even though raw meat retains more nutrition, it seems that it may be a bit more difficult to digest than meat pre-digested with heat. So, with raw meat you are getting more nutrition but assimilating less and with cooked meat you are getting less nutrition but assimilating more. With this in mind, here are some preparation ideas to get the most nutrition out of your animal protein.

When you cook your meat, cook it as lightly as you can possibly stand so the inside flesh is on the raw or rare side. Searing a few seconds to a few minutes on each side is an excellent method. This uses heat to kill off any bacteria on the outside of the flesh while preserving the amino acid and heme iron content of the meat that wasn't affected by the heat on the interior. If you don't like it that rare, then cook it a little longer to medium rare but no more.

If you just can't handle the rare meat qualities then you can try the "slow and low" method. Cooking at low temperatures over a long period of time such as in a crock pot, slow cooker, or roasting pan is also a good way to preserve nutrition and prevent the formation of harmful by-products. Sashimi is an excellent way to get those raw fish proteins and steak tartare and eggnogs are other great ways to get the natural raw animal proteins. As a note: don't ever eat raw hamburger or raw poultry unless you were the farmer and the butcher and you are incredibly clean in your butchering and packing methods.

What about parasites and other bacteria? Well, what does Nature do about these critters? It is important to understand that these organisms are a natural part of life and we are endowed with mechanisms to protect us against them. Our first defense mechanism is our own digestive juices! A pit of hot bubbling acid! That is how wild carnivores kill off the bacteria they ingest... haven't you wondered why they don't get sick from eating road-kill?

Parasites are a fact of life, we all have them (some of us have more than others). We want to keep them at bay by keeping our immune systems strong and healthy. This is done by following the path of Nature as you've been reading in this book. These parasites, whether actual worms or bacterial imbalances, can also be eliminated by taking corrective measures with herbal cleanses. You de-worm your doggies and kitties right? Why de-worm you and your family? You will learn more about cleansing and detoxification soon.

Scavengers and the Unclean

As an aside, there is a reason the ancient Biblical text warns against eating certain types of animals.[12] These fall into either being predatory animals which are carnivorous or animals who are scavengers. Animals which eat other animals are higher up the food chain and concentrate toxic chemicals more than animals which eat plants alone. Because of this, don't eat bears, cougars, birds of prey such eagles and owls, or dogs or cats. (Does that require much convincing?). Don't eat reptiles like tortoises, crocodiles, snakes and lizards or other creepy-crawlies. (Unless you just want to do it to say you did!) Don't eat fish without scales or fins like sharks, eels, marlin, swordfish or any fish that are high up on the food chain or which scavenge for their food like catfish, carp, or suckerfish.

Don't eat other animals that scavenge for their food and eat garbage. This group includes pigs, crabs, lobsters, shrimp, clams, oysters and other shellfish (these are just too tasty, though, not to have once in a while if you like). With respect to the chemical contamination found in tuna and other fishes, that subject will be saved for the Day 9 chapter on fats and oils. Finally, it's probably just sound advice to completely avoid disease-carrying rodents like mice, bats, rats, rabbits, squirrels, weasels, ferrets, raccoons, skunks and moles. (Just in case you were thinking about inviting the neighbors over for some barbecued mole... Nummy!)

The bible also warns against eating the blood or the fat from an animal. The fat is where fat-soluble nutrients can be stored but it is also where fat-soluble toxins can reside. It is impossible to avoid fat when you consume the meat of animals but it would be wise to avoid their *concentrated* fat. You want to avoid a big mouthful of petrochemicals or solvents or pesticides if you can. The physical rationale for not consuming animal blood is less clear, although on a spiritual level, it is the considered to be the life force of the animal and not to be eaten. Blood is very high in mineral and protein nutrition but it would also be high in waste products which would otherwise be filtered by the kidneys and excreted.

So that is that. Basically add an appropriate amount of animal protein, even if it is a single bite, at each meal. Amino acids are the building blocks for every blood cell, brain cell, heart cell, bone cell, immune system cell... you name it. It is vitally important to eat this animal protein to get the full range of amino acids and minerals and vitamins which are not found in plants alone. After you are in this protein routine for several months, you may feel like you want to take a break from eating meat so often. That is okay, it is important to listen to your body and follow its wisdom. Go ahead and cut it back- just don't eliminate it entirely. You would follow the same sample menus (back of book) with the appropriate servings of starch and veggies and just cut out the protein for an occasional meal.

START TODAY:

- Include some protein from an animal source at each main meal. The amount would be approximately 3 ounces of raw or cooked animal protein per meal for a person with average digestion.

- If you tend to the vegetarian type body then focus on meats which are lighter, such as fish, chicken, turkey and other fowl, and eggs. The amount would be approximately 2 ounces of animal protein per meal. If you are not ready for animal protein yet, just start with a few ounces of broth to get the body accustomed to it.

- If you are more the carnivorous type, you would be better off with richer darker, fattier meats such as those found in oily fish, the dark cuts of poultry, duck, goose, red meat of all types including wild game and free-range organic grass-fed beef. The amount would be approximately 4 ounces per meal.

Summary: This is what I'm doing up to this point, each day adds onto the next

Day 1: **Food awareness:** Keep a diary of my foods. I am accountable.

Day 2: **Water:** Sip half my body weight in ounces throughout the day.

Day 3: **Movement:** Some exercise performed every day. Note it in my diary.

Day 4: **Regular meals:** Eat about the same time each day.

Day 5: **Vegetables and Raw Living Foods:** 50% of total weight of your food.

Day 6: **Fruit:** Up to 2 servings of locally grown fruit daily (no fruit juice)

Day 7: **Carbohydrates:** One serving per meal combined with vegetables.

Day 8: **Protein:** One serving of healthy animal protein at every meal.

Choose only free-range organic or wild animal proteins.

The average person should consume about 3 ounces per meal.
Some may need more or less depending on the criteria mentioned.

MAMMALS	POULTRY	FISH	CAUTION: *only occasionally*	DO NOT *even* THINK *of it...*
beef *free range or grass fed organic*	chicken	anchovy	catfish	bat
buffalo	cornish hen	bass	clams	bear
elk	duck	caviar	crab	cat
goat	goose	cod	lobster	cougar
lamb	pheasant	grouper	mussels	dog
moose	quail	halibut	octopus	dolphin
organ meat *(liver, heart, etc)*	turkey	herring	oyster	eagle
rabbit	EGGS	mackerel	pork	lizard
venison		perch	scallops	mice
		rockfish	shrimp	mole
		roughy	squid	owl
		salmon	tuna	raccoon
		sardines	ahi	rat
		snapper	mahi	shark
		trout		skunk
				snake
				squirrel
				swordfish
				turtle
				whale

- PROTEIN -

[1]"Primate," Microsoft® Encarta® Online Encyclopedia 2009
http://encarta.msn.com © 1997-2009 Microsoft Corporation.

[2]An R Acad Nac Med (Madr).1998;115(2):397-413; discussion 413-6.Comparative study of the administration of anabolic amino acids. Confirms the discovery of the Master Amino Acid Pattern] Lucà-Moretti M

[3]It is estimated that humans began cultivating food for agricultural purposes about 10,000 years ago.

[4]J Nutr. 1998 Oct;128(10):1716-22. Digestibility of cooked and raw egg protein in humans as assessed by stable isotope techniques. Evenepoel P, Geypens B, Luypaerts A, Hiele M, Ghoos Y, Rutgeerts P.

[5]Comp Biochem Physiol A Mol Integr Physiol. 2007 Nov;148(3):651-6. Epub 2007 Aug 16. Cooking and grinding reduces the cost of meat digestion. Boback SM, Cox CL, Ott BD, Carmody R, Wrangham RW, Secor SM

[6]Br J Nutr. 1994 Aug;72(2):221-41. The effect of heat on amino acids for growing pigs. Van Barneveld RJ, Batterham ES, Norton BW.

[7]Journal of Food Science Volume 48 Issue 4, Pages 1366 – 1367

[8]Heat treatment on heme iron and iron-containing proteins in meat: Iron absorption in humans from diets containing cooked meat fractions The Journal of Nutritional Biochemistry, Volume 7, Issue 1, Pages 49-54 M.Garcia, C.Martinez-Torres, I.Leets, E.Tropper, J.Ramirez, M.Layrisse

[9]Carcinogenesis. 1984 Jan;5(1):95-102. Isolation and characterization of new mutagens from fried ground beef. Felton JS, Knize MG, Wood C, Wuebbles BJ, Healy SK, Stuermer DH, Bjeldanes LF, Kimble BJ, Hatch FT.

[10]Princess Takamatsu Symp. 1990;21:279-88. Heterocyclic amines produced in cooked food: unavoidable xenobiotics. Sugimura T, Wakabayashi K, Ohgaki H, Takayama S, Nagao M, Esumi H.

[11]National Cancer Institute. 15 Sep 2004. http://www.cancer.gov/cancertopics/factsheet/Risk/heterocyclic-amines

[12]Leviticus 7 22-27, Leviticus 11

Day 9
Fats, Oils, & Dairy Products

FAT. A word that brings up an undesirable feeling and association for most people. In fact, many of you chose to read this book because FAT has become an all too familiar part of your life. In actuality, yes, most people are living a life of dietary excess. Especially because most people reading this book are from countries where food is abundant and fat is a characteristic ingredient of the food we eat which gives it incredible taste and texture.

Fat though, is not always a bad guy. Have you heard the term "essential" fatty acids? Well, that is how important fat is; it is essential and vitally important for the functioning of your body. It exists in the structure of every single cell keeping it strong and resilient. Fats are important for your glandular health and for keeping your hormones in balance. They play a key role in reducing inflammation which means less pain and less chronic disease. Fat makes up about 60% of the dry weight of your brain and that is fat we couldn't do without! (Remember, a hydrated brain is about 80% water so these two substances are vital for healthy brain functioning.)

It is with choices of the kinds of fat eaten where most people go wrong. Too many of the wrong types of fats consumed for too many years, as delicious as they may be, add inches to your waist, put plaque in your arteries, and knock the healthy fats in your cells out of balance. Heart disease, stroke, diabetes and cancer could all be dramatically decreased if our food choices did not include these bad fats.

So what are the best fats for our bodies? Again, we have to look to Mother Nature and follow Her lead. In Nature, fats and oils are not separate from the other nutrients with which they are packaged. Do you know of any plants which are secreting droplets of oil ready to be dipped with bread or drizzled on your salad? Certainly not! Instead, plants provide oils in a ready-to-eat package called a nut or a seed. Alternatively, we may also consume fat from animals when we eat their muscle. Both sources of fat are found in Nature combined with plant or muscle fiber and protein. In Nature, fats and oils are never found in forms independent of protein and fiber.

It is important realize that even oils considered to be healthy are not natural. Fish oil, flax oil, nut and seed oils are also not natural. These oils have been processed to remove the oil from the natural protective fibers of the nut or seed. The unprotected oil is now susceptible to the exposure of air, light, and heat. Oil exposed to these elements can easily become rancid or can oxidize. Oxidation is the chemical reaction in which fat molecules lose electrons. Electrons are healthy charges which can neutralize toxins in the environment. Losing electrons, the fat becomes a dangerous free radical and instead of protecting against toxins it becomes a toxin itself. Free radical oxidation is a cause for premature aging. None of us needs assistance in getting older!

Even the "cold-pressed oils" can oxidize unless they are kept out of the light and heat and are consumed quickly. It is better to stick to Nature's perfect package and eat the whole fish, the whole nuts, and the whole seeds, raw and unprocessed. Research indicates that the beneficial omega-3 fish oils are better absorbed when eaten in the form of the whole fish as opposed to swallowing fish oil capsules. People who eat fish as opposed to swallowing pills see a 25% greater increase in their EPA levels.[1]

Not all Fats are Created Equal

Fats come in many different chemical varieties with names like saturated fats, mono-unsaturated fats, poly-unsaturated fats and cholesterol. Saturated fats are commonly tagged as the bad guy because they are found mostly in meat and dairy products. Scientists also thought at one time they may be the root of all evil and the cause of heart disease, but modern research is suggesting that these fats may not be the guilty party after all. Saturated fats are more rigid because they are "saturated" with hydrogen atoms.

Mono-unsaturated fats are considered neutral fats. They are high in foods like olives and olive oil, avocadoes, macadamia nuts, peanuts and other nuts, and seeds. They have been helpful in balancing the "bad fats" in your blood. These oils are a liquid at room temperature and become solid when chilled.

Polyunsaturated oils, or polyunsaturated fatty acids (PUFAs) are always liquid because they are not saturated with hydrogen atoms. They are broken into two families: the omega-6 and the omega-3 oils. The omega-6 family of oils includes alpha linoleic acids (LA) and gamma linoleic acids (GLA). Alpha linoleic acids occur in high concentrations in corn, soybean, safflower and canola oils. As you'll see, Western diets tend to be already too high in these oils. These oils were once considered to be healthy, but no longer. Replacing butter with margarine is proving to have been a disaster. Gamma linoleic acid shows up in borage seed, evening primrose seed and black currant seed. GLA is quite helpful in alleviating symptoms related to the imbalance of hormones which often accompanies PMS and menopause.

Polyunsaturated fats of the omega-3 family include the oils alpha linolenic acid and EPA and DHA. Alpha linolenic acid (ALA) is a fatty acid found in high amounts in flax seeds. In a healthy body, ALA can be converted into EPA and DHA, which are the activated oils beneficial for health. The highest natural sources of EPA and DHA are found in fish and in breast milk. These valuable oils are consumed by a baby when it breastfeeds and help make a healthy brain and nervous system. They also keep the cardiovascular system healthy and can reduce pain and inflammation.

Let's not forget the fat which is commonly considered the bad guy: cholesterol. We'll talk about him in a moment, and we'll see if he is really so bad after all or if he has been falsely accused of cardiovascular crime.

Fats in Nature have vital purposes. Your nerves and your brain are made almost entirely of fats. Fats also are what the body uses to build the majority of your hormones, especially sex hormones. Fats are used to make hormones called prostaglandins that send messenger signals for pain and inflammation. Are you in need of a vital boost to your memory? Are you lacking libido or sexual desire or is your performance poor? Maybe you are in chronic pain? Good fats play a vital role in supporting the health of these areas.

Fat Shifters

Fats provide support and structure to the cells of plants and animals, keeping the good stuff in and – hopefully - the bad stuff out. Some cells are more fluid-like and some are more rigid depending on the proportions of different types of fats in their membranes. A cell which has more cholesterol and saturated fatty acids will be more rigid. A cell which has more unsaturated fatty acids will be more fluid. As an illustration, a stick of butter high in saturated fat and cholesterol is solid while vegetable oil, which is high in unsaturated fat, is liquid.

A plant or animal will have different compositions of fat depending on the environment in which it lives and the foods it eats. Different fats have different freezing and melting points; for example, if a certain oil becomes too cold, it can "freeze" and become hard and clumpy. You may have seen this happen if you have put olive oil in the fridge and it clouds and becomes more solid. On the other hand, if you put olive oil in a pan on high heat it will become very liquid. Miraculously, plants and animals can change the ratios of fatty acids in their cells to adapt to the conditions of the environment. If the cell becomes too rigid or too liquid, the cell could die.

For example, plants or animals living in colder climates will produce fats which stay liquid at cooler temperatures so the fat doesn't become too rigid and kill the cell. In warmer climates, plants and animals will produce fats which are more rigid so the oil will not become too liquid and kill the cell. Coconuts which are grown in warmer climates have a higher content of rigid saturated fats than coconuts grown in cooler climates. Nuts or seeds which are grown in cooler climates have a higher content of slippery unsaturated fatty acids than those grown in warmer climates.

Fish can also change the content of their cells depending on the temperature of their environment. Organisms which live at lower temperatures have more unsaturated fats in their cells than the same organisms living in warmer temperatures.[2] It is fair to say then if you want to eat higher proportions of healthy omega-3 oils in your fish then you will want to purchase fish caught from the cold waters closer to the North and South Poles.

The fat content of animal flesh also changes, depending on the foods they eat in the wild or what they are being fed commercially. Red meat from beef has been a big source of controversy for many years. Often we hear that saturated fat and the resulting cholesterol will kill, and it might very well do just that if it is present in excess. The problem partially lies in our gross over-consumption of these rich meats and also in the quality of the animal meat we are consuming.

Farmer Fred or Mother Nature

The meat you are eating from most grocery stores and restaurants is NOT NATURAL. These animals raised on farms are fed very differently from animals that feed in the wild. Animals in the wild run free and have a varied diet high in nutrition. Wild game animals such as turkey, deer, elk, moose and buffalo have incredibly healthy meat, which is lower in saturated fat and cholesterol. These animals are not penned up and injected with chemical hormones and antibiotics like their cousins raised in a feedlot. They eat mostly grass, plants, shrubs, berries, leaves and tree branches high in healthy omega-3 fats. When the animal eats these plants, these good fats concentrate in their tissues. When you in turn eat these naturally raised wild animals, these healthy fats get transferred to your body's cells.

Conventionally raised beef is quite different. This is the beef that you eat at restaurants or purchase from the grocery store. These cows are raised in crowded concrete, dirty, mucky, manure-filled feedlots where they never have fresh green grass below their feet on which to graze. Instead, they are fed a diet high in corn, soy, or other grains so they can be fattened to maximize their weight. (Hopefully the beef you are eating was not fed ground up body parts of other cows which can lead to, among other things, mad cow disease). A wild cow would never have a diet of concentrated oily grains or unnatural foods. Wild cows would not be wallowing in their own poo all day nor would they be hunting other cows as food. Does that sound like the kind of conditions from which you'd want your meat to come?

An animal in Nature would not be sitting on syringes filled with growth hormones to artificially mature it. An animal in Nature would not need to be shot up with antibiotics so it can survive the diseased and inhumane conditions it endures in the crowded feedlots. You must understand that these chemicals, and many others with which these animals are being mediated, are transferred to your body and your children's bodies when you eat them! We should not support this method of farming. Instead, we must encourage the production of meat that is good for the environment, good for the animal, and good for our bodies. Please watch the movie *Food Inc.* for a look at how the meat you are eating is really produced.

Farmed meats in general are not as healthy as animals from the wild because most farmers do not raise animals in a health-conscious manner. Farmed chickens are given feed containing hormones and antibiotics as opposed to free-range chickens who get to scratch the dirt and pick at the bugs. Farmed chickens are kept in wire cages and forced to live in the most horrendous crowding conditions. The stench of ammonia from their own excrement burns their lungs and puts them at risk for disease. The eggs and meat from these birds is like eating robot chicken clones.

The Legendary "Fish Story"

Fish that are farmed have the same disadvantages. They are fed food that makes them higher in unhealthy fats. In some cases, the nutritionally deficient fish food causes the flesh of the fish to become so anemic and gray that red dye is added to it to turn the meat pretty pink again. I guess the farmers realized it was harder to sell fish which had "gray" meat.

Farmed fish are also more likely to accumulate toxic chemicals like Polychlorinated biphenyls (PCBs) due to the farming conditions under which they are raised. Even the journal Science warned that farmed salmon contain 10 times more toxins like PCBs and dioxin than wild salmon.[3] In Nature, fish meat and the oils it contains are an ideal health food. Add humans to the equation and we figure a way to cut corners which evidently seems to screw it all up. When in doubt, go without. Unless it is for a special occasion or at a special restaurant, do not eat or buy farmed fish for you or your family.

Heavy metals found in wild fish are an impending health catastrophe and something of which we need to be aware. Mercury is the biggest concern, especially for women who are pregnant or want to become pregnant. It is considered one of the most toxic non-radioactive substances on earth! Mercury is a very strong inhibitor of neurological function and can be damaging to a developing brain AND a mature brain. We need to wake up as a world community and stop polluting our food!

We have not been good stewards of our land. Our waters are full of waste from factories and burning fossil fuels and from our carelessly dumping household chemicals and medications down our drains. The mercury and other contaminants from these substances flow from our drains into the streams into the rivers into the oceans and it is absorbed by the plants. The little fishes eat the plants and the bigger fishes eat the little fishes and finally we eat the bigger fishes with all this concentrated mercury poison. We are literally poisoning our own food supplies and contributing to our own demise!

Animals higher up in the food chain should be avoided for this reason. This includes predatory and large fish like shark, swordfish, marlin, ahi, mahi, and the favorite TUNA! The U.S. government advises pregnant women and children not to eat more than one serving (4 ounces) a week. Why would you want to eat even one serving if you knew there was a chemical in it which could harm you or your baby? I highly recommend watching the academy award winning documentary of 2010 titled, *The Cove*, which highlights not only the dangers of mercury poisoning but also the yearly slaughtering of thousands of dolphins in Japan killed for food. Dolphins and whales are too high up the food chain and concentrate dangerous toxins; they should never be consumed.

If you choose to take the risk and eat tuna anyway, it should only be eaten in the "chunk light" form as opposed to the "albacore." These are smaller tuna that do not grow as large so they do not accumulate large amounts of mercury. Do your best to avoid mercury by buying wild fish from clean cold Northern waters. Choose fish which are lower on the food chain, especially the tiny fish of sardines, herring, and mackerel. Remember to avoid the meats and fish listed as "unclean" from Day 8 because of their high position on the food chain or their propensity to eat garbage.

Back again to the meat. "Where's the Beef?" Well, it is hidden between all those layers of FAT. That's what you get when animals are fed with all this excess grain and corn. You create an animal that produces the most beautiful marbled steaks filled with fat that just sizzles on the barbeque and just melts in your mouth... tender and delicious! Mmmm good! If you have ever been to a country which is less economically advanced and you order a steak from a local diner don't be surprised if it is chewier and less flavorful. It is actually better for you, because it was raised in the back yard on grass and weeds. It hasn't been fed the fat and oil from the grains to give it that juicy marbling for which customers pay a premium price.

We are very naturally attracted to fatty foods. It is our survival genes that attract us to foods high in fat. We desire it because it is a high-energy food and higher energy meant that we could survive another day. Our ancestors never knew if they would have food one day to the next so it was important to be able to sniff out the highest energy food. In fact, people who are carrying more fat have stronger survival mechanisms than those people who are skinny. Their genes are literally more protective in times of famine; their ancestors were able to store the food they ate more effectively than those who didn't. Those survival genes really came in handy when we lived off Mother Nature, but are not so useful anymore now that there is an abundance of food, all filled with FAT!

The Fat Outlaw

So what about cholesterol? That is a bad fat, right? Well, actually, not as bad as you've been told. Cholesterol is manufactured by the body for many vital reasons. Did you know that cholesterol is used by your body to make your hormones like DHEA, testosterone, cortisol, estrogen, progesterone and vitamin D? What would you do without those? So cholesterol isn't bad per se; it can be a problem when the bad cholesterol outweighs the good cholesterol.

So why is the cholesterol there in the first place? Aside from the functions already mentioned, the body uses cholesterol to heal itself. Think of cholesterol as little band-aids the body is creating in response to an injury. Yes, your body is amazing; it even has its own band-aid company! So you really have to ask not how to get rid of the cholesterol, but how to get rid of the injury. Injury is represented by inflammation. Actually, you are already on your 9th day of reducing inflammation through diet, water and exercise. (In my next books, we'll talk about reducing inflammation caused by stress.) By adopting the changes discussed in this book, you will be amazed not only by the improvement in your cholesterol values, but in the improvement of all your bodily values which are influenced by inflammation.

Cholesterol comes in two forms: the so-called good HDL or "healthy" and the not-so-good LDL or "lousy." When your tissues become damaged through inflammation, cholesterol is made for repair. If your body makes too much LDL (lousy cholesterol) and it becomes oxidized or damaged then you have the beginning of a vicious cycle. These oxidized or damaged LDLs can then cause the destruction of the arteries leading to atherosclerosis and heart disease.[4] LDL can be damaged by free radicals from chemical toxins in the environment as well as artificial flavors, colors, preservatives, excess sugar and polyunsaturated fatty acids (PUFAs) found in processed foods. Stay away from these and choose food high in natural antioxidants like vitamins A, C, and E by following Nature's plan. We'll talk more about antioxidants soon.

If oxidized cholesterol can cause damage inside the body who's to say that consuming cholesterol already oxidized can't do the same thing? In fact, it does! Cholesterol's bad rap may not actually be due to the presence of the cholesterol itself but rather to how we are eating cholesterol-containing products. Your bad cholesterol LDL levels can also rise if you are consuming foods high in COPs! (Stop that! Don't think such thoughts!)

Cholesterol Oxidation Products (COPs) are formed when cholesterol-containing foods are exposed to light, air, heat and time which causes oxidation. Cooked or stored foods containing cholesterol form up to 10 times more COPs than raw fresh food containing cholesterol.[5] COPs have been shown to increase LDL as well as promote the atherosclerosis which leads to heart disease and stroke.

They have also been implicated in the creation of cellular mutations leading to cancer.[6,7] If you are eating foods high in COPs by improperly cooking or storing your food, then you are putting yourself at risk. More will be learned tomorrow on preparation.

D-EVIL-ED Eggs

Eating animal foods high in cholesterol, such as eggs, is a very safe and healthy practice when prepared properly and combined with vegetables high in antioxidants. Recent research shows that a person will have no appreciable increase in blood cholesterol levels even when eating eggs daily.[8] This is strong evidence that eating foods high in cholesterol is not the reason we are seeing higher levels of cholesterol in the blood.

Eggs, which are one of the highest sources of cholesterol, have been given a very bad rap since 1909, when a researcher named Ignatowski produced atherosclerosis in rabbits by feeding them a diet of meat, eggs and milk.[9] Hey, I know Easter is a pretty exciting time of year, but I haven't ever seen bunny rabbits eating chick chick eggs (let alone steak and ice cream)! In fact, grass contains absolutely ZERO cholesterol. Does steak and eggs seem like the proper diet for a bunny rabbit? Of course not! Rabbits do not have the mechanisms to process cholesterol like other animals so these studies are not even relevant to humans.

When humans eat eggs in their whole form - both yolk and white - as Nature intended, they are an excellent food. They are high in assimilable protein and are an egg-cellent source of essential fatty acids and vitamins and minerals. Don't separate the yolk and the white; eat them together. Interestingly the cholesterol is better emulsified and digested by the lecithin that is found in the whole egg. Don't over-cook your eggs either; more about cooking eggs tomorrow.

Speaking of not separating whites from yolks, I should make note of a question that patients often ask me: "What about Egg Beaters™ ?" How do you think I would respond to that? That's right, "NO!" The reason is because these are a processed food. The yolks are separated from the whites because of the concern for cholesterol. To repeat: recent studies indicate that eating egg yolks every day does not affect cholesterol. Also, I do not like using Egg Beaters™ because it is made from the eggs of chickens penned up in coops. Again, choose your eggs like you choose your meat: free-range and organic if possible.

The Real Bad Guys Unveiled

You may be surprised to hear that many of your so-called "healthy vegetable oils" are really not so healthy. These fall under that category of Poly-Unsaturated Fatty Acids also known as PUFAs. Some examples are soybean oil, canola oil, safflower oil, and corn oil. Believe it or not even your flax oil, hemp oil, sesame oil, wheat germ oil, and fish oils are all PUFAs and are potentially harmful. These oils are processed with the use of intense pressure, chemicals, and heat to extract them from the plants or animals in which they occur. High heat and chemicals oxidize these healthful oils into unhealthy oils and are more likely to cause heart disease, cancer and many other diseases.

Dozens of studies have shown that these oils are very susceptible to oxidation after processing. They are easily damaged by light and air when they are extracted from the fiber that protects them within the kernel or seed. This means that they are oxidizing when the bottle is opened and white they are sitting on your counter exposed to the air and the light. This oxidation forms free radicals which we already know not only prematurely ages the body but also can oxidize the LDL cholesterol. If this happens, the not-so-good LDL particle becomes a bad particle that can accumulate and lead to heart disease and stroke.

What is more, these PUFA vegetable oils are very high in omega-6 oils and very low in omega-3 oils. Nature's foods eaten by our ancestors consisted of fats with a ratio or 1:1 or *equal parts* of omega-6 to omega-3 fatty acids. Today our Western diets are approximately 16 parts omega-6 fatty acids to one part omega-3 fatty acids (16:1) and this unhealthy ratio has been implicated in imbalance prostaglandins and in the occurrence of pain and inflammation. This elevated ratio of omega-6 to omega-3 is also proven to promote the pathogenesis of many diseases, including cardiovascular disease, cancer, and inflammatory diseases like arthritis, asthma and autoimmune diseases. Studies prove that in lowering the intake of PUFA vegetable oils and increasing omega-3 oils, there have been suppressive effects on these diseases.[10]

Because they can promote health and deter disease, I recommended eating an abundance of foods high in omega-3 oils (See the list at the end of the chapter for healthy natural sources.) In some patients with a predisposition to cardiovascular disease, nerve or brain disorders, auto-immune processes, hormone imbalances, or inflammation and pain, I will often recommend taking a supplement to boost their omega-3 levels. These should be oils purchased in the grocer's refrigerated section in dark glass containers or in capsulated form. These oils should be protected from oxidation by keeping them from exposure to heat and air.

Polyunsaturated fats are being praised for their health-promoting effects, but saturated fats have still not been totally exonerated of the evils of which they've been accused. Saturated fats and cholesterol are high in animal products as well as in breast milk. Would Nature really put something harmful in the food that it uses to nourish a growing baby? Palm oil and coconut oil are two plant oils that are both high in saturated fat. These oils have been used by indigenous tribes for millennia to nourish their people. Interestingly, these oils are now being praised as healthy oils after being vilified for years for their high content of saturated fatty acids. In reality, scientists are thinking that the link between dietary saturated fats and heart disease is not strong, and may be nonexistent. Maybe there is more to the story than what science has traditionally thought?

Clean the Cupboards and Kiss the Cook

There are only a couple of oils that should be considered safe and reasonable to use for general cooking. Olive oil is the great neutral diplomat. If it was a country it would be in a peaceful union with all. It is mostly monounsaturated fat which is a neutral type of fat. It is an oil which can be pressed from the olive without using harsh chemicals or high heat extracting methods. Of course, this is only if you choose the EXTRA VIRGIN OLIVE OIL. If the label says "virgin olive oil" or just "olive oil," don't buy it; it is overly processed. You can heat extra virgin olive oil, but only on low heat. It also makes a great condiment on vegetables and grains or mixed with lemon juice or vinegar for a dressing on salads.

When cooking at higher heat, choose coconut oil or palm oil which have a greater saturated fat percentage and are less likely to oxidize. You can even use a little butter or beef tallow to cook at higher temperatures but make sure they do not brown or "smoke" which increases oxidation potential. These fats can handle the higher heat better than the polyunsaturated vegetable oils (PUFAs) listed above.

You may have heard of ghee which is also called "clarified butter" which means it has the milk protein removed. This has been used widely in India for thousands of years and is a staple in Ayurvedic medicine. You can also cook with ghee on higher temperatures than with butter because the dairy solids have been removed; again you do not want it to brown or smoke. Lard is not recommended because it comes from the fat of pigs which are scavengers and concentrate toxic chemicals in their fat tissues. Beef tallow is cleaner than lard if it comes from an organic source. Extra virgin olive oil is your best choice for an all-purpose neutral oil for cooking on low heat.

Fake Fats

At one time medical science used to warn us against eating butter. They told us to throw it away and trade it for the "heart-healthy" margarine. Isn't it amazing how medical science changes its mind year after year? All they had to do was to look to Nature to find the real answer. Most people now know the dangers of using oils like margarine, and vegetable shortening like Crisco, and spray-on non-stick oils that we at one time thought were a healthy alternative to butter.

These fake fats fall under the umbrella of PUFAs but these are even more dangerous. These are further processed by a chemical process called hydrogenation which turns liquid oil into solid oil at room temperature. These are called hydrogenated and partially hydrogenated fats or you might have heard them called by the name "trans-fats." These fats cause the good cholesterol HDL to drop and the bad cholesterol LDL to rise, making the victim who eats them more likely to develop heart disease. They are now currently associated with multiple diseases like diabetes, obesity, Alzheimer's disease, cancer and infertility. Do not eat food prepared with margarine or vegetable shortening or trans-fats.

It is important to be aware of another gazillion dollar marketing technique used by food processing companies. Are you the individual who buys foods labeled "fat-free," "light," or "reduced fat" hoping that you are saving your family and yourself from the pitfalls of obesity? Unfortunately these foods are not any better for your health than their "full fat" original formula siblings.

These foods still use PUFA oils, although in lesser quantities, and partially replace them with modified starch and sugar; basically they trade the PUFA load for a sugar load. You'll see this commonly in mayonnaise and salad dressings but you may also see it in "fat-free" and "reduced fat" chips and snacks. These often trade out the PUFA oils with the chemical "Olestra™". This is a completely artificial man-made chemical that is synthesized to taste and feel like fat although the body does not recognize it as fat. It is completely unnatural and should be avoided because the long term affects of ingesting this foreign substance are unknown.

Some companies do make health-conscious foods which are legitimately fat-free and they advertise them as such. These are foods which are prepared without extra fats or oils. If the label describes the food as "fat-free" or "reduced fat" and the list of ingredients contains only food from natural sources and no PUFA oils, then you may consider it as a possible food selection. In general though, be careful of food that is marketed as "fat-free."

Do the family a great healthy favor and eliminate all foods with hydrogenated and partially hydrogenated oils and Olestra™ on their labels. With the growing negative press, the fast food restaurants have started to eliminate them and even some governments are passing laws to mandate against them. Hey, if the government is finally doing something about it, it must really be bad: you should get them out of your house, too! Vegetable shortenings like Crisco™ and fake fats like Pam™ and margarine and even those supposed health spreads like Smart Balance™ are not smart! These are not natural foods; they have never been found in Nature and only exist because they were processed by man!

Udderly Unnatural

Speaking of butter, this is a good time to talk about the fat which comes from the udder of cows! Got milk? Not for this program you won't. My grandmother told me that milk is a Bible food and therefore healthy for us. It is true that cow's milk was consumed in Biblical times. It is also true that healthful milk and milk products as they were eaten in Biblical times are no longer readily available. Cows at one time were raised close to Nature, grazing on grass, without hormones, antibiotics or other chemicals.

Milk in ancient times was not pasteurized and therefore it was abundant in natural bacteria which are healthful for our own intestinal landscape. When the raw milk was allowed to age, the naturally occurring bacteria soured the milk and created kefir, yogurt, and buttermilk. This milk also was not homogenized, so the particles of milk were not so tiny that they could pass directly into our circulatory system increasing cardiovascular injury. No other animal species in Nature drinks pasteurized or homogenized milk. This is a processed substance; only we smart humans drink it!

In keeping with the theme of the book, if you are perceptive and look to Nature, you'll observe another very obvious answer. Is there any other animal in Nature which continues to suckle from its mother's breast after it has been weaned? Think hard and you will come to the conclusion. When a baby develops to a certain point, it stops suckling milk from its mother. Can you possibly imagine still suckling off your mother at your age right now? All other animals stop…why don't you? Nowhere in Nature do animals drink milk after they are no longer babies!

Furthermore, is there any other animal species in Nature which suckles from the breast of another species? I have never heard of rats suckling from coyotes or horses suckling from elephants. Why should you suckle from an animal that is a dozen of times larger than you with no resemblance to your own species? The milk of a cow which is higher in fat and protein than human milk was designed to turn a baby calf into a gigantic cow. Milk from a cow was meant to turn a newborn calf into a 150 pound cow in 6 weeks. Does that sound like something you want to feed your baby? It just doesn't make sense for us to be drinking cow's milk. (Even if you wanted to drink milk that Nature made for us, you might be hard-pressed to find a human donor).

Milk was intended to fuel and build a newborn baby into a big baby and then a bigger baby and finally child. Milk is a food which causes babies to grow and it does this rather quickly and it really is Nature's Perfect Food, but it is only for babies. It is an anabolic substance, meaning it makes cells grow and replicate- exactly what is needed for a baby to mature. Do you really want to continue to grow after you have already grown? Not really, because the only growth will be in your pants size! A big belly is neither good for your heart, your brains, nor any other organs. Especially those below the belt!

Booooo the Mooooo

Is there any wonder that America is in the midst of an epidemic of diseases which are anabolic dominant or growth dominant? We eat so many foods that are rich and concentrated putting our cells in an anabolic state. This anabolic dominance causes high blood pressure, high cholesterol, high blood sugar and leads to heart disease, diabetes, stroke and some cancers. Milk, cheese, ice cream, butter and yogurt are very rich anabolic foods and should be saved just for an occasional treat. There are, however, some health conditions for which I will use raw, unpasteurized and non-homogenized milk for patients.

Primarily, I will prescribe it for those special people who are in a very sickened state and not able to put on weight. In these cases of digestive illness, where patients are not able to digest heavier foods, this may benefit them. I especially recommend consuming raw unsweetened kefir and raw unsweetened yogurt. Only in these cases do I recommend consuming dairy products as Nature intended: raw dairy products. Remember that milk does not come from the udder of a mammal in a pasteurized and homogenized form, right?

Goat's milk is no exception; it is milk from another species and unless you want your child to be as big as a goat, or worse, a cow, don't drink it! In some cases, raw goat's milk can be a suitable replacement for children who are unable to breastfeed. Of course, the breast is still best. From birth until the first four to six months, mother's milk should be the sole source of nutrition for the infant.

Only use alternative forms of milk if it is necessary for the child's health.

Milk, butter, cream, cheese, ice cream, yogurt and yes, milk-chocolate all fall into the category of dairy and they are not foods Nature intended for us to eat after we are weaned. It doesn't mean you can't enjoy a nice ice cream treat on a summer's day or a delicious slice of pizza once in a while, it just means you shouldn't eat it regularly. The same goes for butter; use it as a treat, and cook with it when olive oil or coconut oil are not available. Even though non-dairy creamer is labeled as "non-dairy," it is actually made from the protein of milk, casein. Its ingredients include vegetable oils, sweeteners, and artificial flavorings and colorings; stay away from it, too.

So, where then are you supposed to get your calcium if it's not from milk as the TV commercials want you to believe? Well, it is important that big business stays in business by persuading you to buy their products. Those commercial advertisements telling you that "milk does a body good" and that milk is needed to provide calcium for your bones, is effective marketing and advertising. It is paid for by the Dairy Council of America to convince you to buy milk for your health. The truth is, if you don't buy milk, the people of the dairy industry will need to find other professions. We will cover more on calcium when we get to minerals but for now let's ask this: "Where does a cow get its calcium?"

Fast Track to Fine Fats

The finest way to increase these good oils is in the whole food form. Choose to add more good fats from nuts and seeds and dried meats and fish and eggs, all of which are excellent snacks. They have no sugar and are high in good quality protein and fat nutrition. The raw nuts and seeds make great snacks to nibble on in place of your sweet snacks. They really settle the munchies and the oral fixation as well as sugar cravings. Raw means they are not roasted, deep fried, or salted. If you are an average sized person used to moderate activity and you notice yourself getting hungry between meals you may choose to have a couple handfuls of raw nuts and seeds or a serving of any of the other suggested snack ideas a couple times daily.

A complete list of snack ideas will be listed in the menu planner in the back of the book.

It is especially healthful to incorporate the use of raw nut butters like almond butter, sunflower butter, and peanut butter which make great snack dips for celery, carrots and apples. Sometimes taking a spoonful of nut butter plain can be a great way to calm a sugar craving. Be careful with too many nuts and seeds if you are someone who gets herpes breakouts. Nuts contain a higher amount of the amino acid arginine than lysine and can cause viral herpes breakouts in susceptible people.

What about your salad dressing and mayonnaise without which you think you can't live? Instead of buying your salad dressings pre-made, it is easy to concoct your own from scratch using extra-virgin olive oil, apple cider vinegar or lemon juice, spices and sea salt. You can even make your own mayonnaise from extra virgin olive oil as instructed by the Nature's Diet Cookbook. (see Sources)

You can put the healthy oils on your vegetables or grains to give them added flavor for your meals. The whole idea is to move away from foods which are high in PUFA vegetable oils such as bleu cheese, thousand island, or ranch salad dressings and mayonnaises and switch to extra virgin olive oil. If you just can't live without these dressings, try diluting your favorite salad dressings 50/50 with olive oil. You can do the same thing with the butter you can't live without. Melt a stick of butter on low, add an equal portion of olive oil, stir together into a mixture and put it in the fridge to solidify. This way you are getting just half the quantity of PUFA or butter at one time because it is diluted with extra virgin olive oil.

[1]Lipids. 2006 Dec;41(12):1109-14

[2]Environmental and metabolic animal physiology By Clifford Ladd Prosser pp125-136

[3](Science jan 2004)

[4]Libby P. Inflammation and cardiovascular disease mechanisms. Am J Clin Nutr. 2006;83(suppl):456S-60S. Tontonoz P, Nagy L, Alvarez JG, Thomazy VA, Evans RM. PPARgamma promotes monocyte/macrophage differentiation and uptake of oxidized LDL. Cell. 1998;93(2):241-52.

[5]J Agric Food Chem. 2004 Aug 11;52(16):5290-6. Links Effects of different cooking procedures on lipid quality and cholesterol oxidation of farmed salmon fish (Salmo salar). Al-Saghir S, Thurner K, Wagner KH, Frisch G, Luf W, Razzazi-Fazeli E, Elmadfa I.

[6]Annals of Clinical and Laboratory Science, Vol 19, Issue 4, 225-237 The role of cholesterol oxidation products in the pathogenesis of atherosclerosis RJ Morin and SK Peng

Summary: This is what I'm doing up to this point, each day adds onto the next

Day 1: **Food awareness:** Keep a diary of my foods. I am accountable.

Day 2: **Water:** Sip half my body weight in ounces throughout the day.

Day 3: **Movement:** Some exercise performed every day. Note it in my diary.

Day 4: **Regular meals:** Eat about the same time each day.

Day 5: **Vegetables and Raw Living Foods:** 50% of total weight of your food.

Day 6: **Fruit:** Up to 2 servings of locally grown fruit daily (no fruit juice)

Day 7: **Carbohydrates:** One serving per meal combined with vegetables.

Day 8: **Protein:** One serving of healthy animal protein at every meal.

Day 9: **FAT:** Eliminate bad fats and add one serving of good fat per meal.

[7](Arteriosclerosis, Thrombosis, and Vascular Biology. 1998;18:1885-1894.) Arterial Injury by Cholesterol Oxidation Products Causes Endothelial Dysfunction and Arterial Wall Cholesterol Accumulation James X. Rong; Shanthini Rangaswamy; Lijiang Shen; Ravi Dave; Yi H. Chang; Hazel Peterson; Howard N. Hodis; Guy M. Chisolm; Alex Sevanian

[8]Barraj, et al. A comparison of egg consumption with other modifiable coronary heart disease lifestyle risk factors: A relative risk apportionment study. Risk Analysis. Published online November 4, 2008.

[9]Anitschkow N, Experimental Arteriosclerosis in Animals. In: Cowdry EV, Arteriosclerosis: A Survey of the Problem. 1933; New York: Macmillan. pp. 271-322. AND Steinberg D, The Cholesterol Wars: The Skeptics vs. The Preponderance of the Evidence.2000; San Diego: Academic Press.

[10]Biomed Pharmacother. 2002 Oct;56(8):365-79. Simopoulos AP. The importance of the ratio of omega-6/omega-3 essential fatty acids.

START TODAY:

- Today start by reading labels and become aware of the types of fats in your foods that are not natural. See the following table to see the good, the bad, and the uglies.

- Clean out your cupboards by throwing away all foods with bad fats (and artificial ingredients). Be careful not to purchase foods that have the ingredients on the bad or ugly list. Stay away from fast foods and junk foods which will most likely contain high amounts of these unhealthy fats.

- If you are an average-sized person who engages in moderate activity you can start today by either adding a 15 gram serving of oil listed as "best" or "good" in the table below to each meal. This will be about 1 tablespoon (15 g) of oil or fat or about 2 tablespoons (32 g) of nut or seed butter or about 3 ounces (84 g) of fresh avocado added to each meal. You may also eat a couple handfuls of raw nuts and seeds a couple times daily as a snack.

- If you consider yourself overweight or you want to lose weight, then add 1-2 teaspoons (5-10g) of healthy oil or nut or seed butter per meal. You may choose instead to have one ounce of fresh avocado per meal. You may eat only a single handful of raw nuts and seeds a couple times daily as a snack. Better snacks for those trying to lose weight will be those which are high in vegetable fibers like carrots, celery or other vegetables dipped in hummus or bean dip.

- If you are an athlete or if you are underweight then fat will need to be your friend. Fat is Nature's storehouse for energy and you will need to increase your intake if you are expending a lot of energy or not putting it on. Increase your fat up to 2-3 tablespoons (30-45 g) per meal of healthy oil or 3-5 tablespoons (48-80g) of nut or seed butter per meal or 6-9 ounces (168-252g) of avocado per meal and even more if you are working out extremely hard or are severely underweight and need to maintain body weight. In addition choose to snack on high fat raw nuts and several handfuls of seeds between meals.

The average person will consume about 15 grams of fat per meal which is about one tablespoon of oil or about 2 tablespoons of nut or seed butter.

BEST	GOOD (keep from air, heat, and light)	BAD (too high in omega 6: omega 3 ratio)	UGLY
extra virgin coconut	black currant seed	canola	butter flavored oils
extra virgin olive	borage oil	corn	hydrogenated oils
raw nuts seeds/ butters	evening primrose	cottonseed	margarine
almonds	fish oil	safflower	mineral oil
cashews	flax oil	soybean	Olestra™
chestnuts	hemp oil	sunflower	partially hydrogenated oils
coconuts	krill oil	Smart Balance™	petroleum based oils
filberts	palm oil		spray non-stick oils
flax seeds	peanut oil		trans-fats
macadamia	sesame oil	lard (pork)	Crisco™
pecans	walnut oil		Pam™
peanuts	wheat germ oil		
pine nuts	butter		
pistachios	ghee		
poppy seeds	tallow (beef)		
pumpkin seeds	(raw dairy)		
sesame seeds			
sunflower seeds			
walnuts			
olives			
avocado *3oz.*			
coconut milk *2oz.*			
fish serving *100g = 2500mg EPA = 8 capsules fish oil*			

Day 10
Preparation, Cooking, & Portion Size

Besides knowing what to eat, you will also need to know how to eat it. The key to eating healthy is being self-sufficient since it is nearly impossible to find restaurants offering the healthy choices Nature intended.

The biggest complaint I hear from my patients when they are making healthy lifestyle changes is, "I just don't have enough time to eat this way." This is certainly a real dilemma and I understand it completely. Eating well, although it is simple, really does require more time than going through the drive-thru or having the delivery man show up with a pizza or some Chinese food. As with anything else, there is a learning curve involved. Although healthy food requires some preparation time, once you develop a system you'll see it doesn't take much more time than other foods. Besides, the rewards you gain- health, slimness, and a youthful and energy-filled body are well worth the extra minutes a week.

Another misunderstood idea is that healthy food is more expensive. That is a valid concern considering the current state of the world's economy. Healthy food for your family should not have to break the bank, and actually, when you live according to Nature, not only will it NOT break the bank; it's one of the most economical ways to live.

"Tuppence a Bag"

Whole foods ideally are just that: foods prepared by Nature and ready for us to eat. In an ideal world, the food Nature offers us would be primarily raw, fresh and ripe from the vine. Because our lifestyles no longer allow for this we want to come as close as possible to this model. Much of the expensive processing done to make foods look, smell, and taste better is not in harmony with Nature. And as you have probably noticed, prepared foods are also THE MOST EXPENSIVE foods available. This is due to the costs the company incurred to pay for that big manufacturing plant with all those employees and the many costs associated with packaging, marketing and shipping those products. And as with any form of production, those costs are passed along to the consumer. That food company takes all those natural whole food ingredients and turns them into something that resembles food but with the added punch of flavor and color to which your senses have become addicted.

Don't be fooled by the processed foods coming to us in packages, cans and boxes even if they happen to be sold in a health food store with the label reading "natural" or "organic." There can be some healthful alternatives to your junk food out there, but for the most part, they are nevertheless what can best be considered "healthy junk food" because while they utilize good ingredients they are still processed foods. If you desire these healthy junk foods as a treat once in a while that is fine, but don't create a dietary staple out of them. The processed foods found in health food stores are by far some of the most expensive of all! This is where many people get the mistaken idea that health food is expensive. People see the prices for the ultra-healthy veggie pizza or vegan lasagna or the whole-grain organic chocolate cookies or the dairy-free frozen treats and go "HOLY EGGPLANT, that is expensive"! Your right; it IS expensive. In fact, it is actually just very expensive processed food that has a healthy twist, and still not what Nature intended.

Stop buying ready-made or prepared foods in packages, boxes and cans. You will not only save money on your bills, but you will also save space in the landfill. Preparing your own foods means you create less waste from less packaging material and in the process you are helping the planet as well as yourself and those for whom you cook.

Choosing organic foods would be ideal, but for someone on a budget they are not an absolute must. Buy organic where it is an affordable alternative. Meat and meat products are the most important foods to purchase as clean as possible. Do not buy meat unless it is wild game, organic, free range or it is raised by your local farmers chemical-free. Meat is high on the food chain and can concentrate toxic chemicals at high levels. If you eat meat high in hormones, pesticides, antibiotics and hundreds of other poisons, they will be transferred to your body. Organic meat is no doubt the most expensive part of any diet but what extra you spend here can and will be saved in what you spend on produce and bulk foods.

It's a Whole New World

Many healthy foods can be purchased for your family at a far lower price in the produce and bulk foods sections of your market. When shopping in the produce section take the food lists from Day 4- Day 9 and try every item that you have not tried before. Why not? Because you never know; you might really like it! In order to be successful with natural foods you have to branch out and try as many new foods as possible to add variety. Go ahead and make a special date to spend a few hours at the grocery store. Make it fun and shop like you have never even been in a grocery store before. This time, shop with a whole new outlook and curiosity, taking note of all the new options available to you from these lists. Try as many new foods as you can to expand your palate and provide more variety and more nutrition.

While in the produce department, select primarily those foods which are in season. If you don't know what's in season, ask your grocer. It would be best if the food wasn't imported because those countries' standards for fertilizers, pesticides and herbicides may not be at healthful levels. If you don't know how to prepare it but you've always wanted to try it, BUY IT! It is so easy to look up ways to prepare eggplant by simply typing "eggplant recipes" into the internet search. You might be pleasantly surprised on how easy and inexpensive it is to eat fancy and tasty foods for little money. Impress your partner, your family and your friends!

Produce is one of the fastest foods to spoil and most of us do not know how to store it properly to maintain its longevity in the refrigerator. Plants naturally give off a gas called ethylene which causes them to ripen. In fact much of the fruit that is picked unripe is shipped to your grocer green and then gassed artificially with ethylene prior to being put on the shelf to ripen there. The phrase "one bad apple ruins the whole bunch" is due to the high amount of ethylene gas being released from the bad apple causing the others to spoil quickly.

The best way to store your produce is to remove the vegetables from the plastic bag, wash them, and place them in the crisper drawer in the fridge. If that isn't available, leaving the plastic bags in the fridge is okay as long as the bag is open and not tied in a knot or sealed. You may also put a little bit of water in the base of the bag as well to keep the vegetables hydrated. As long as there is an opening for the ethylene gas to escape and enough water for the veggies to remain crisp, they should stay fresh for a week. Tupperware containers are also fine for a short time, but vegetables stored in them are more likely to spoil due to accumulating ethylene gas.

Another place in which to expand your culinary horizons is the bulk foods section. Here you'll find grains, beans, nuts and seeds of many kinds. There are also lots of other tasty things here, such as granolas, trail mixes and chocolate covered raisins, but use discipline and keep your hands out of those bins for the present! The bulk foods section is where you can get more bang for your buck; a lot of food for a good price. These dried bulk foods when cooked expand to amounts much larger than they are in the dried form. You can literally buy enough food to feed an army for the same amount of money that you would spend feeding your family with prepared or restaurant foods.

How does one even know what to do with those bulk foods? It is easier than you think. Just dig in and try 'em out! Go ahead and buy some grains, some beans, lentils, split peas, whole grain pastas and anything that is on the food lists at the end of the chapters for Days 7 and 9. Try a little bit of anything you haven't eaten before. Take it home and again, if you don't know how to prepare it, Google it! Also, Nature's Diet Cookbook is a meal planner with recipes to help you learn how to prepare some of these new foods. There are literally thousands of recipes out there and all you want to do is get a taste and see if it is something you like or not. Once you decide on the grains or beans that you really like, your next step will be to buy them in larger quantities and experiment with different recipes.

A Crock of What?

A great money and time-saving technique is to invest in what is called a slow cooker or crockpot. This is an excellent way to prepare food for yourself or the entire family with ease. It is also proving to be one of the healthiest ways to cook. Research is proving that when you cook your food "slow and low," you are preventing toxic by-products from being formed during cooking. To cook in a slow cooker, simply add your lentils or split peas or beans or grains along with some fresh vegetables, some water or broth, spices and little sea salt and just plug it in. Come back home ready to eat a fully prepared meal after work or the next morning. It is as if you had your own personal cook busy at home while you were working! It is really so handy and convenient, and there are many slow cooker cookbooks from which to take recipes that will add variety to the diet and keep the family happy.

Another nice thing about slow cookers is that large quantities of food can be prepared at the same time. Leftovers are a wonderful way to eat healthy by simply reheating the food from the day before. Or if you want more variety, simply freeze that which is unused and reheat it later in the week. Shopping in bulk and cooking in bulk means there is always an abundance of food available at a very affordable price.

While on the subject of the slow cooker, it is not only excellent for making soups and grain and bean dishes but also for cooking meat. Remember cooking slow and low is one of the healthiest ways to prepare meat. It is so delicious and handy to put in a whole chicken and throw in some potatoes or rice along with some onions and garlic. Just plug it in and 6 hours later, a beautiful bird is ready to eat! Cooking in quantity is the key and you can do the same with a roast or whole fish. Cook up a large quantity and you'll have enough for the whole week. You will also have enough for snacks when you get hungry, and you can even put some in the freezer to have weeks later. The more you prepare at one time the easier meal preparation will be for the remainder of the week. Simply enough, pull off a chunk of meat, a scoop of this grain or lentil or potato, add a few handfuls of salad and voila! Out the door! You can prepare a full and healthy meal literally in minutes and it is more beneficial to your body and to your pocketbook than any restaurant alternatives could ever be.

While we are still in the bulk foods section, don't forget to try some of the raw nuts and seeds. Raw simply means they are not roasted, deep-fried, or salted. The raw nuts and seeds make great snacks through the day in place of sweet snacks and they really settle the munchies and the oral chewing fixation as well as defeat those awful sugar cravings.

Awaken the Slumber

A note here about beans, legumes, grains, nuts and seeds - these are all considered to be seeds themselves. If these seeds are planted and watered they will sprout and make new plants. The seed itself is high in the nutrients which are needed by the sprout for energy until it can grow roots and get its own nutrition from the soil. This seed is dormant when we eat it, but we can actually activate the life of these seeds when we soak them in water. This will turn them into live plants. By simply soaking dried beans, legumes, grains, nuts or seeds in water overnight, and rinsing them afterwards, you have changed the properties of the food. It has been changed from a dormant grain to a living plant made up of activated living cells all filled with nutrition.

Nature brings a mature seed to life when it is dropped from the plant into the soil. When the rains come (which is the soaking), the seed swells and enzymes are activated to signal the plant to sprout. The seed is transformed from a sleeping food to a LIVING food and if eaten raw (such as the nuts and seeds) you are ingesting a food which is more digestible and vital with living cells and activated energy. Doesn't eating a live food just sound healthier?

If you have extra time and energy you can take the soaked seeds from above and place them on a sprouting tray to sprout and then prepare food from them. There are several companies which actually sell sprouting baskets or kits. When you eat sprouts, you are eating food which has different chemical properties than the original seed. This sprout is now a live plant which is consuming the starch that was present to get the plant started and is full of living cells with activated enzymes, vitamins and minerals.

If you are going to cook beans at home, you may want to follow these ideas to remove as many of the gassy gas molecules as possible before eating them. Remember the magical fruit they are! Some people will do well with beans which are soaked overnight then rinsed and cooked. Other people are so sensitive to them that it requires another step to remove more of the gassy molecules. After beans are soaked overnight, discard the water, rinse and then cover them with water one more time and quickly bring to a boil. Once they boil, take the pot off the heat and discard the water again. Rinse these flash-boiled beans again and now you have the beans which are ready to be cooked for your meal. Because the gassy molecules are water soluble they will dissolve in the flash boiled water and can be rinsed off easily. Do not add salt or acids like vinegar or tomato too early in the cooking of the beans; some people feel this will make the skins tough. Consider adding either of these after the beans are cooked.

Rare, Medium, and Well Done

Regarding cooked foods in general, let's review a few important factors discussed previously. First, cooking has not always been natural for humans and it is not at all natural for animals. To be in accordance with Nature as much as possible, it is important to eat an abundance of raw foods, especially if you are healthy and have a strong digestive system. Cooked food is favored over raw foods for people with digestive weakness or if there is a need to sterilize against bacterial or parasitic contamination.

Vegetables are best if kept raw and alive. If they are to be cooked then steam them lightly so they maintain their bright colors and firm crisp texture. You do not want them to be soft, colorless, brownish or mushy. Vegetables are also good to stir-fry in a pan with a little olive oil, coconut oil, or even plan water or broth. Again, do not cook them too long or they will get mushy. If you are cooking several types of veggies at once, put the firm ones such as carrots in first and then the soft ones like spinach later.

Do not boil your vegetables unless you are boiling them in water to make a soup. Of course, soup is an excellent way to preserve the goodness of vegetables because the nutrients lost in boiling will be absorbed into the soup's water which will then be consumed with the rest of the soup. Soups are excellent ways to get good, healthy, nutritive foods into people who have weak digestive systems or are young, elderly, weak or ailing.

As for cooking with oils, remember that the oils which can best tolerate heat are coconut oil, palm oil, tallow, ghee, and to a lesser extent, butter. These oils handle higher heats without being changed into chemical forms that can be dangerous and potentially unhealthy. Do not use soybean oil, corn oil, canola oil, safflower oil or any other type of oil listed under "bad" or "ugly" from Day 9 because they do not handle the heat well and oxidize into unhealthy chemicals. Extra virgin olive oil is a good all-purpose neutral oil and you can also cook with it on low heat. If you are following Nature's path you wouldn't choose butter as a staple but it is not a problem to use it occasionally for special dishes.

The starches in your meal, such as the grains, rice, corn or potato, are best cooked in a slow cooker or even in a rice steamer. You can also try roasting corn or potatoes on a grill or baking them in the oven. You can also cook your grains the old fashioned way - in a pot on the stove. Carbohydrates are long chains of sugar molecules linked together. The longer they cook, the more easily they will be digested in the body, so it is preferable to cook carbohydrates well so they will be digested completely. In Nature, we would be eating them raw or sprouted, but for modern convenience we will eat these cooked.

Meats are best kept in their truest natural form – yes, RAW! (or at least as close to raw as possible). Nature's animals aren't barbecuing their steaks and we shouldn't be either. Meat which is cooked lightly or kept somewhat rare is the best way to preserve the nutrients like amino acids and vitamins while eliminating any bacteria that may be on the exterior. Because we are not eating it directly from the freshly butchered animal, there is a higher chance of bacterial contamination. These bacteria are not necessarily harmful as humans have eaten fermented and rotten meat for millennia, but it just may not settle too well on our ultra-sensitive tummies.

I recommend that you sear your meat very quickly in a hot pan for a few seconds to a few minutes, depending on the meat. You want to maintain the quality of the meat as much as possible by keeping it as rare as you can on the inside. Call it rare, extra rare, or BLUE if you are a savage! This is fine for steaks, especially with free-range organic meat or if it is prepared in a good quality restaurant.

Be much more careful with poultry like chicken and turkey cooked on the rare side. If you know the source and you trust the cleanliness you can also cook them on the more rare side. You'll notice how much more tender the poultry is by not cooking it to a leathery texture. I would not suggest eating hamburger raw unless it is ground from clean steak which you prepared by yourself on the spot. Raw hamburger can have bacteria growing within the patty itself.

If you don't like rare meat, you can use the slow cooker or rotisserie to make the cooking of poultry and roasts easy and efficient for the family. Cooking "slow and low" in a crock pot or roasting at low temperatures are also excellent ways to preserve nutrition and prevent the formation of harmful by-products.[1] If you cook slow and low you do not need to eat the meat rare because the dangerous byproducts are kept to a minimum. You may lose some essential nutrients but in exchange the protein will be pre-digested by the heat.

Grilled by COPS

Barbecues are a catch-22 because they can taste "oh so good" but leave behind that charcoal residue which has been proven to cause cancer and other disease. Maybe another signal from Mother Nature that raw meat is better than cooked? If you are using a grill, sear the food and do not overcook it. Grilled veggies do not concern us as much as grilled meat because the heat does not form dangerous chemicals in them the same way.

Remember that grilled meats form chemical by-products (polycyclic aromatic hydrocarbons (PAHs) and heterocyclic amines (HCAs)). In addition to grilling and barbecuing, you should also be cautious about frying and broiling meat. These methods of cooking produce the largest amounts of HCAs because they are cooked at very high temperatures for long periods of time. Be very careful not to order your meat well done or "charred" because it is loaded with PAHs and HCAs. Another helpful way to cut your risk of consuming HCAs is by marinating your meat in Nature's antioxidants. Herbs, spices, and fruit extracts of all types have antioxidants that protect against dangerous chemicals. Research has shown that an olive oil, lemon juice and garlic marinade as well as red wine and other herbal marinades cut HCA levels in chicken by as much as 90%.[2]

Eggs would also be best if they were raw or if they are poached, soft-boiled, or lightly fried. Absolutely no scrambling! Scrambling an egg breaks the yolk on the hot pan causing the cholesterol to oxidize. Remember the COPs? No, not the red and blue flashing lights which make your stomach rise up into your throat on the freeway. The Cholesterol Oxidation Products that are formed when you eat foods that contain cholesterol exposed to high heat. These COPs are considered big players in atherosclerosis and the cell mutations seen in cancer. We don't want any COPs in your eggs! That crispy brown coating that forms when eggs are cooked with too high of heat is loaded with COPs. This is not good. Do not eat it.

Instead of scrambling your eggs, fry them lightly by putting a little olive oil in a pan on medium heat, crack a couple eggs, and cover them with a lid. The water from the eggs will evaporate and steam the top of the egg. You can choose the desired consistency from runny to firm depending on the time they are allowed on the heat. And do not overcook hard-boiled eggs. You do not want the yolk to be hard, green and crumbly. Instead bring your eggs to a boil, turn off the heat and let them sit 15 minutes and then cool them down with cold water. The yolk should be creamy inside.

Preparing food for minimal exposure to high heat or cooking food "slow and low" are the best ways to avoid these chemical by-products. Research shows that the highest levels of COPs are formed when foods containing cholesterol are pre-cooked and then reheated.[3,4] In other words, ALL PACKAGED AND PREPARED FOODS containing cholesterol are much more damaging than food you prepare yourself! Do your best to avoid prepared food. This may be one of the biggest causes of disease in countries which consume high amounts of restaurant food, fast food, and frozen foods which require reheating.

Are you still hung up on not scrambling your eggs? Well then, maybe you'd like to try eating your eggs as animals do in Nature. In short: Rocky Balboa style! Rocky had it right: Crack the egg, and GULP! Down the hatch raw! Slip slidin' down the gullet! Try it yourself and make a home-town eggnog. Take two or three organic free-range eggs, blend them with a little rice milk or almond milk and flavor it with a little cinnamon if you wish. Then, down the hatch! This can make a great morning breakfast, a light snack, or a great workout protein drink. It is also good for folks who are recovering from illness or are unable to chew properly. Recipes for this protein drink and other meals listed in the menu plans can be found in the Nature's Diet Cookbook.

If you are going to eat your eggs raw buy ONLY organic free-range eggs grown by a farmer whose chickens live in the open grass and scratch at the soil to feed on the minerals and bugs. These are healthy chickens getting nutrition from Nature as it was intended. Eggs from healthy free-range farm chickens are the only eggs you can safely eat in their raw form. Concerns about salmonella are mostly for those eggs from chickens cooped up in the most unnatural state of wire chicken factories. In these coops the chickens live crowded together in deplorably dirty conditions with their beaks cut off to keep them from pecking the other chickens. They are injected with hormones and antibiotics to keep them growing and to prevent them from contracting diseases in their terrible living conditions. These are definitely not the birds you want to provide you with their eggs or their flesh!

Again, Nature has no way to cook its food, so all animals living off the Earth eat food that is raw, unaltered by heat. As we know, humans are the only animals who eat cooked food. Although there are advantages to eating cooked foods, there are also serious disadvantages. Cooking pre-digests food but it also destroys amino acids, vitamins and essential nutrients. Cooking can also form some dangerous by-products which can be carcinogenic. Keep this in mind so you can prepare your food to maximize the good qualities and minimize the bad ones.

Savor the Flavor

If you want to add extra flavor and nutrition to your soups, beans or grains, try making your own bone broth from the leftover meat bones. Take your chicken, turkey, or beef bones (even try oxen tail and chicken feet) after they have been picked of the meat and put them with water in your slow cooker, pressure cooker or even on the stove in a pot to boil. If you are cooking these on the stove bring them to a boil and then turn it down so they can simmer for hours. You want to boil them long enough so that the bones themselves can be somewhat broken down with a potato masher after several hours. Not all the bones will break down but the small soft ones will disintegrate after a while. You want the broth to turn a whitish grey. This liquid is pure nutrition.

After the bones have broken down, strain off the broth from the bones and pour into a tall jar. You will see the fat will rise to the top after a bit of time. Skim off the fat and throw it away. Now you have a beautiful bone broth that can be used to cook all your grains and soups in place of water. You can even add a little salt and seasoning and drink it straight! It's delicious and these bones are loaded with the nutrition you need to make your bones strong as well. It's a fine source of calcium and other bone-building nutrients just as Nature intended. Recipes made with the bone broth will be found in Nature's Diet Cookbook.

This is a good time to discuss something we LOVE - our sauces and dips. In fact, many of you can't even eat vegetables without these dips. I have found it to be a struggle to find healthful alternatives that taste as good as the sauces and dips we love. Many of these are made with mayonnaise, canola oil, or other vegetable oils which are loaded with unhealthy PUFAs. Or they might be full of high fructose corn syrup and other sugars, like the ones found in ketchup and barbecue sauces. To make matters worse, they are often flavored with artificial flavor enhancers like MSG and tainted with artificial colors and preservatives. Maybe these addictive chemicals are precisely why we love to dip and dunk any food we can in this stuff.

Instead of buying your sauces, dressings and dips, try to make your own at home. You can make your own mayonnaise-based dressings and dips from the home-made olive oil mayonnaise as found in Nature's Diet Cookbook. You can also make salad and vegetable dressings from extra virgin olive oil, apple cider vinegar or fresh lemon juice, spices, and salt. Easier yet is buying dressing packets from the store and simply adding the recommended ingredients. I highly recommend the company Simply Organic™ for a wide assortment of dressing and condiment mixes (see Sources). You can also make your own toppings like fresh guacamole, bean dips, hummus and salsa. (see Nature's Diet cookbook for recipes)

If it is just too much to ask of you to make such changes so quickly try this method. Split your favorite salad dressing 50/50 with olive oil if you really can't quite say goodbye to it. This will make it not quite so unhealthy. Remember that you can also do this with butter. Organic ketchups, barbecue sauces, and mustards can be found at health food stores although the taste may take some getting used to. Be especially careful with these sweet sauces if you are diabetic or trying to lose weight.

Use only natural sea salt or mined mineral salt because they have no additives or chemical enhancers. I like Celtic Sea Salt™, Redmond Real Salt™, and Himalayan Pink Salt™, to name a few. These natural salts are usually grayish, brownish, reddish or bluish in color, which is a sign the salt contains healthy trace minerals. These are minerals not found in standard chemical table salt, which is simply sodium chloride. Because they have no additives, these natural salts will also have a tendency to clump. All herbs are excellent for flavorings as are the herbal powder seasonings that are sodium-free such as powdered kelp, Mrs. Dash™ or Spike™. Some spices like black and red peppers can be too harsh for people with delicate systems, so use them wisely.

Rogue Receptacles

So what are the best materials in which to cook? Glass is very good to cook with because it does not allow metals to leach into the food like some types of pots and pans. Make sure your pots and pans are made from GLASS or STAINLESS STEEL and NOT ALUMINUM. If you don't know ask someone. Aluminum is a metal which over the course of time can be absorbed into your food from the heat of cooking. It has been proven that high aluminum levels can increase the rates of Alzheimer's disease and certain cancers. Throw those pans into the recycling bin, and don't even give them to anyone else or they could be poisoned, too. Aluminum is so potentially toxic that you should also make sure that you do not drink from aluminum cans or use underarm antiperspirants with aluminum. Aluminum toxicity has been shown to be associated with neurological diseases like Alzheimer's and Parkinson's diseases.

And throw away any of the NON-STICK frying pans. They are made with a chemical which is poisonous to humans. This chemical is a form of Teflon that has been linked to birth defects, hormonal imbalances and cancer. Again, choose glass or stainless steel and add a little bit of oil on the pan to make sure the foods don't stick. As mentioned on Day 9, DO NOT USE PROCESSED NON-STICK SPRAY OILS EITHER! These are chemical oils and should not be used to make food easier to remove. They oxidize with heat and are associated with various health problems.

Plastic bottles, containers, bags and wraps are drowning both us and our planet. Plastics are man-made artificial chemicals and when they get into your body they can – and do - adversely affect your health. Research is proving that plastic molecules are responsible for birth defects, hormonal abnormalities in men, women and children, immune suppression, auto-immune disease and cancer. Your body doesn't recognize plastics because they are not natural. Keep them out of your food by doing your best not to eat anything which has been stored in anything made from plastic. This is especially important with fatty foods like meat, butter and cheese. If you do store food in plastic or plastic bags be sure to first wrap it in wax paper so the food doesn't directly touch the plastic. This includes wrapping your children's sandwich in wax paper before putting it in the sandwich bag for their lunch.

Because plastics can be melted by heat, never warm up food in plastic- period. When plastic becomes warm, the molecules speed up and are deposited in the food with which they come in contact. This is very dangerous situation. Do not heat food in plastic bags, Tupperware or other types of plastic containers. When in doubt, go back to the old reliable containers made of glass or stainless steel. And here is another reminder: try not to drink water stored in plastic. Be especially careful of any fluids which have been sitting in plastic bottles in the sun! You do not want to be ingesting these toxic chemicals. If you need reminding, go back and re-read the information about water and plastics in Day 2.

Catch the Waves

Convenience cooking has been simplified greatly by the discovery of the microwave oven. Today it is common to find microwaveable dinners in plastic trays sold in the frozen-food section of your market. Beware: these can be a time-saver, but they can also be a time bomb for your body! Of course, these are ready-made processed foods and as such, are filled with artificial chemicals, flavor enhancers and preservatives. Add that chemical load to the combination of cooking it in plastic AND by the heating effect of radiation waves from a microwave, and WOW! Ka-Boom goes the toxic explosion! And SCREAM go your cells!

Microwave ovens emit microwaves which are a form of "non-ionizing radiation." This type of radiation is generally considered "safe" because it hasn't been shown (yet) that eating food cooked this way is damaging to humans. Non-ionizing radiation comes in the form of radio-frequency energy, visible light waves, infrared waves, and microwaves used for cooking and cell- phone communication. The other form of radiation is called "ionizing radiation" and is proven to be dangerous. This form of radiation has enough electromagnetic energy to strip electrons from atoms and cause cellular damage to your tissues. Gamma rays, X-rays, and ultraviolet rays from the sun are forms of ionizing radiation that can cause great harm to your body.

Sunlight also emits microwaves but these are in the form of direct current (DC) versus the alternating current (AC) emitted from the microwave oven. The radiation from a microwave oven causes the molecules in the food to rotate millions of times per second in an alternating current which results first in friction and then heat. Because the microwave forcefully rotates polar molecules in the food, the surrounding molecules can be damaged by being torn apart or deformed. Production of free radicals and mutant molecules like isometric amino acids is a likely result of this forceful rotation. What is the ultimate effect? Well, it is hard to know definitively at this point. There is limited research on the long-term effects of microwaved food on human health, but microwave cooking has been shown to cause the same nutrient losses as other forms of cooking. It has also been shown to form more COPs when cooking chicken as compared to chicken which is pan fried.[5]

Microwaves are convenient but their use should be limited as much as possible. As in other forms of cooking, the longer and higher the heat, the more likely it is to cause unfavorable reactions. Reserve the microwave oven for quickly warming something up for a small amount of time but do not use it often. It is better to heat something on the stove, in the oven, or even in a mini countertop toaster oven with radiant heat than to expose it to microwaves. Until we understand more on heating with microwaves versus traditional radiant heat, we should choose what is closest to Nature.

While we are on the topic of radiation, there is a new form food sanitation that is coming to a grocery store near you: IRRADIATION. The word itself doesn't sound healthy and this new method of sterilizing food is bound to be controversial in the near future. Irradiation utilizes ionizing radiation (the harmful type) called gamma radiation to kill bacteria which spoils food. The ionizing radiation not only kills the bacteria but it also removes electrons from the food you are about to eat. This creates dangerous free radicals.

This process also can create new toxic by-products in the food: compounds such as benzene, formaldehyde and lipid peroxides are known to cause cellular damage and mutations when ingested. Gamma radiation is powerful and can inactivate a high percentage of the available nutrition including antioxidants, vitamins and amino acids. There are not enough long-term studies to determine if this form of sanitation could eventually cause cancers and other diseases. Be careful of any food labeled with the words "electronic pasteurization," "pasteurization with X-ray" or "cold pasteurization" which are all synonyms for IRRADIATED FOOD. Be cautious and steer clear.

Beat the Buzz

This is a small detour but while we are on the subject of frequency and radiation and microwaves let us further discuss those bands of unseen energy swirling all around us like cosmic dancers. What we can't see can't hurt us, right? More like…out of sight out of mind! We would rather not know than to have to worry about it now. This attitude could have deadly consequences in the future. We should be aware of the significance that cell phones and these EMF (electromagnetic frequency) microwaves and radio frequencies have had on our health since their use has become widespread.

The cell phone is a very convenient tool. We wonder how we ever managed without it. In many ways our lives seem simpler with them but at the same time more complicated than ever. Your day is now filled with people who are easily able to call or text you at any moment of the day or night, cluttering your thoughts with their problems and dilemmas. Think about how dramatically email changed the nature of communication. Now instead of receiving a hand-written letter once a month you receive many electronic message in a single day, all of them clamoring for a quick response. When was the last time you wrote or received a hand-written letter? Is your life really that much simpler with email and cell phones?

Multiple studies suggest that the use of these devices emits waves that may cause harm in those whose brains are still developing. If the studies reveal harm to anyone with living cells, shouldn't we be sufficiently concerned to consider what they might be doing to all of us? Yes we should! If they can harm a child, they can harm all of us on some level; we don't yet know to what degree this is happening. Human cells can even be damaged by non-ionizing radiation if they are exposed to these radio frequencies and microwaves for a long enough period of time. Radio frequencies can heat human tissue just as microwaves heat food. Our nerves and glands are especially sensitive to this frequent exposure.

We have to be smart with cell phones and not let children in their teens or younger use them without a headpiece. The headpiece would best be one that had an air communication tube as opposed to a wire or radio. An example would be the "BlueTube™" air tube headset rather than "Bluetooth™". It is a better idea yet to use the hands-free speaker module to keep all electrical components away from the head. Keeping the phone away from the head and out of pockets is important. You want to make sure the EMF waves are not affecting the cells in the brain or the hip bones or sex organs. Every cell functions through electromagnetic frequencies, and frequencies from cell phones can confuse the frequencies your cells utilize for cellular communication. We do not clearly understand the long-term effects of these exposures and must use our best judgment based on the information we currently have.

The young are as obsessed with their texting as they are with their video games. Statistics show attention deficit disorder (ADD) and hyperactivity have hit all-time highs. These mental activities over-stimulate the brain and nervous system. They can stimulate areas in the brain which are responsible for hyperactivity and suppress areas that make a person calmer and more focused. We have to be as aware of the stimulating effect EMF waves have on the children's cells as we are of the effects that texting and video games do.

On a more extreme note, some scientists are even speaking up and predicting that we may be facing a food shortage if the honeybee populations are not rescued. In their important role as Nature's pollinators, honeybee populations are now having a difficult time surviving. The reasons are as yet unknown, but some experts theorize that it may have to do with the growing number of microwaves emitted from cell phones; waves which interfere with the bees' ability to find both food and their homes. If this continues, food could become less available as pollination by the honeybees becomes more difficult.

Preserve or Reserve

Let's return to food. Is it okay to eat frozen or canned foods? Well, that is a toss-up. Remember, these methods of preserving are most definitely NOT NATURAL. Nature preserves food by drying. However, convenience is important, and for that reason it is worth mentioning certain foods which can be better appreciated in canned or frozen form than others.

In general, canned foods do not have the vitality that live foods do. Open a can of green beans, put them side by side on a plate with freshly steamed green beans, and tell me which one looks more appealing. The colors tell you that the steamed food is higher in nutrition and higher in vitality. The one advantage of some canned foods is they are usually picked when they are ripe. Because they are unable to be shipped to the grocery store without spoiling, they are canned at their peak. What you get is a food which is higher in mineral nutrition and bioflavonoids because it spends more time ripening on the plant.

Tomatoes are a perfect example. Canned tomatoes, tomato sauces and tomato juice are actually very good foods which can be used as a base in many soups, sauces and other dishes. They are an excellent source of nutrition when they are picked ruby red, full of the antioxidants lycopene and carotenoids, both of which are known as cancer preventers. They don't come close to resembling their anemic neighbors on the grocery shelves with their pale salmon color. In this case, canned tomatoes are a better choice nutritionally than the raw, under-ripe varieties found at the store. Choose to can your own tomatoes in glass or buy the cans that are lined if you can find them. Tomatoes are acidic and can cause the regular non-lined tin can to leach metals from the can into the tomatoes.

Other good choices for canned foods are meats and fishes. They are a quick fast addition to any meal needing a protein boost and the bones are often cooked with the meat. The bones infuse the meat with calcium and soften to the point where they can be eaten right along with the meat. Eat the whole thing - meat and bone! It is pure nutrition for your body. Think how the carnivorous animals get their calcium; again not from milk! Choose meat and fish that are canned in water, not oil.

I also suggest to people who do not have the time to soak and cook beans to purchase them canned. Canned lima beans, pinto beans, kidney beans, black beans or garbanzo beans make a quick meal for someone on the run. I recommend straining the beans of the fluid they are canned with and rinsing them with water before cooking or eating.

Frozen vegetables such as peas, carrots, beans, broccoli and corn are all fine to add to meals but freezing is not the ideal way to preserve these vegetables. They are especially good to add to a soup or a stir-fry when you need to save time on the shopping, cleaning, and cutting but they are not as good as the real fresh deal because the freezing, just like the cooking, changes the quality of the plant itself. The same as excess heat destroys the living functional enzymes of a cell, so does the low temperatures of freezing. The plant is no longer able to provide your body with the vital activated nutrition you would receive from a fresh, live raw plant. And not only is the plant broken down by freezing, it also gets further broken down by the heat of cooking. The minerals will be maintained but many of the vitamins and amino acids will have been sacrificed. For this reason, avoid these vegetables unless you're pinched for time.

Since drying is Nature's way of preserving food, what about that? Drying is excellent. All the grains and beans and seeds are all stored dry by Nature. When they are soaked in water, Nature activates them and wakes them up for Life. Dried foods should not be eaten dry, but actually in the form that Nature would provide, i.e. reconstituted with water. Dry beans and grains, of course, are best soaked and cooked. Nuts and seeds are best soaked overnight before eating and dried veggies and meat can be put into soups to reconstitute them.

Dried fruit should also not be eaten without soaking it over night- that's right, not even raisins. Dried fruit is too concentrated in its sugar content and is really more like a candy. Fruit, remember, is consumed conservatively, but if you do eat it, do not eat it dried. Adding a few dried raisins and raw almonds to whole grain oatmeal can be a nice treat and a great way to eat dried food.

Eat Like a Cow

Step away from the preparation and consider the amounts of these delicious foods we should be eating. We already covered recommended quantities of the proteins, carbohydrates, and vegetables in the prior chapters. Here are a few more tips that make it even easier to follow those suggestions. First, research has proven repeatedly that the lower our caloric intake, the longer and healthier we live. In fact, there is nothing to date that proves to have a better effect on longevity than cutting back the total number of calories consumed. Of course, cutting back calories means you will be cutting down on the inches and the pounds, too. You can apply this information in one of two ways: you can either eat less or you can eat food which contains fewer calories.

Because vegetables are so low in calories, your transition to a predominantly vegetable-based diet means you will you need to eat more like a cow and graze all day long. When you eat a lot of vegetables, you will be able to feel as if you are satisfying the stomach's need to feel full, and you will also verify the research which says you need to eat fewer calories for a longer life. Can you believe that you can literally eat *a pound of lettuce* and it has approximately the same number of calories as *a single BITE of milk chocolate*?? Is that crazy impressive or what? This is very important because you don't have to starve to extend your life and shrink your waist. You can feel fully satisfied and still follow the path of Nature. Actually, you can go ahead and stuff yourself until you are ready to burst. As long as you are stuffing yourself with vegetables, go ahead and stuff away. Research suggests the result will be a longer and healthier life.

Have you ever noticed that if you go too long without eating you will eventually stuff down so much food you feel as if you could explode? This should no longer be happening to you if you are following the suggestions on Day 4 and eating regular meals throughout the day. You don't want to become excessively hungry. This hunger causes the hormones to become unbalanced and keeps you from maintaining a good weight. Avoid this by eating regular meals.

If you do get overly hungry before a meal, practice moderation and try not to vacuum down the food all at once. Instead, chew a small amount of food slowly and deliberately focusing all your attention on the taste and feeling of each bite in your mouth. By eating a small amount of food and walking away, you'll be surprised how satisfied you are in about 20 minutes. It doesn't take long for the nutrition to hit the blood stream and start satisfying the feelings of hunger. Ever notice how the appetizers that come before the meal satisfy your cravings on their own? By the time dinner arrives, the appetizer has hit the blood stream and your main course isn't nearly as appealing. What if you took this same approach with every meal?

Another trick you can use to reduce your caloric intake is in using different sized plates from which to eat. Choose for each meal a large dinner plate and a small saucer plate. On the small saucer serve the protein and the carbohydrate portions. These foods are more concentrated and higher in calories. Fill the large dinner plate with as many vegetables you wish from the list. You can even fill it again a second or even a third time! This will insure that your caloric intake is not being exceeded and you are staying on track to have a long and healthy life.

START TODAY:

- Go shopping! Go into the grocery store like it is the first time you have ever stepped inside one before. Go into the natural foods section, the produce department, and the bulk foods department and just browse and shop till ya drop. Try, try, try: a little of this, a little of that, and experiment with new recipes and you will come up with many foods that will be friends in your new life.

- Start today by locating a slow cooker or crock pot and buying at least a couple pieces of healthy cookware made of stainless steel or glass, not aluminum or non-stick coating. You must have the tools to prepare your food properly and many of these can be purchased very cheaply at second-hand stores like Salvation Army or Goodwill.

- Try soaking nuts and seeds and beans the night before you eat or cook them and even consider investing in a sprouter to bring them to life.

- Vegetables are best eaten raw, stir-fried, or lightly steamed. Starches are best cooked completely. Meat is best prepared "slow and low" or flash seared on both sides. Marinate any meat that is going to be cooked at higher temperatures or grilled. Eggs should be lightly fried or soft-boiled or even consumed raw in eggnog.

- Enjoy flavor with homemade bone broths made from beef and poultry bones. Make your own dressings, dips and sauces as instructed in Nature's Diet Cookbook.

- Do not store your food in plastic bags without a wax paper liner and absolutely no cooking in plastic containers.

- Avoid cooking with microwaves and avoid buying food which has been sterilized with radiation. Be aware of the electromagnetic frequencies all around us, especially that from cell phones.

- The only good canned foods are tomatoes, beans (such as kidney and pinto) and meat. Frozen vegetables can be used in soups and stir fries but fresh is always better. Drying foods is one of the best methods to preserve the nutrition in foods, but don't eat dried foods without reconstituting them in liquid first.

- Eat regular meals. Take care not to get too hungry between your meals or you may overeat. Eat slowly and deliberately; give your food time to enter your bloodstream. Eat a small amount as an appetizer and see if you are still hungry before eating the rest of the meal. Eat your food from two plates, a dinner plate and a saucer. Pile veggies on the dinner plate and keep the other foods on the saucer.

Summary: This is what I'm doing up to this point, each day adds onto the next

Day 1: **Food awareness:** Keep a diary of my foods. I am accountable.

Day 2: **Water:** Sip half my body weight in ounces throughout the day.

Day 3: **Movement:** Some exercise performed every day. Note it in my diary.

Day 4: **Regular meals:** Eat about the same time each day.

Day 5: **Vegetables and Raw Living Foods:** 50% of total weight of your food.

Day 6: **Fruit:** Up to 2 servings of locally grown fruit daily (no fruit juice).

Day 7: **Carbohydrates:** One serving per meal combined with vegetables.

Day 8: **Protein:** One serving of healthy animal protein at every meal.

Day 9: **FAT:** Eliminate bad fats and add one serving of good fat per meal.

Day 10: Grocery shopping, food preparation, condiments, and serving sizes.

[1]Journal of Food Science, Volume 48 Issue 4, Pages 1366 – 1367 Published Online: 25 Aug 2006

[2]Effect of beer/red wine marinades on the formation of heterocyclic aromatic amines in pan-fried beef. J Agric Food Chem. 2008 Nov 26;56(22):10625-32. Melo A, Viegas O, Petisca C, Pinho O, Ferreira IM.

[3]1: J Food Prot. 2003 May;66(5):840-6.Combined effect of cooking (grilling and roasting) and chilling storage (with and without air) on lipid and cholesterol oxidation in chicken breast. Conchillo A, Ansorena D, Astiasarán I.

[4]Formation of cholesterol oxidation products (COPs) in animal products. Food Control, Volume 18, Issue 8, August 2007, Pages 939-947. S.J. Hur, G.B. Park and S.T. Joo.

[5]J Agric Food Chem. 2003 Sep 24;51(20):5941-5. Consequences of microwave heating and frying on the lipid fraction of chicken and beef patties.Echarte M, Ansorena D, Astiasarán I.

Day 11
Food Combining

How is everything coming along? Are you still writing in your food and exercise diary? Are you still drinking water and including an abundance of vegetables with each meal? By now, you should be starting to notice a difference in how you feel when your body is being cared for the way Nature intended. Let us continue today with more information on how to consume foods properly through their preparation and in the appropriate combinations.

Proper food combining is based on the science of digestion in the human body. It is important to understand that our digestive system produces different digestive juices to break down different types of nutrients in our food. The salivary glands in the mouth, upon chewing, secrete a very alkaline enzyme that breaks down carbohydrates. The first step in digestion begins with this physical breakdown of the food by chewing and mixing and mashing it repeatedly with saliva.

When you swallow the food it goes into the pit of the stomach where a hot bubbling caldron of acid is waiting to break down the food into liquid. Here, the protein is broken down into smaller peptide molecules. As this food moves out of the stomach into the small intestine, it once again meets the alkaline digestive enzymes which are secreted by the liver and the pancreas.

The gallbladder secretes bile which is produced by the liver to help emulsify and break down the fats in your food. The pancreas adds the finishing touches as it secretes the enzymes lipase, protease, and amylase which further breaks down fats, proteins, and carbohydrates. You may think of the pancreas as the organ which keeps your sugar levels in balance, and this is true although it is primarily an organ of digestion. A small number of pancreatic cells secrete insulin and glucagon for blood sugar balance while the majority of the cells secrete digestive enzymes.

In Nature, food doesn't come separated from the sum of its parts. You are not going to find a plant that makes a grain from just carbohydrate molecules alone or a nut from just fat molecules. Food from Nature comes in a perfect package, in perfect ratios of carbohydrate, protein, and fat all ready to be eaten.

With this in mind, you may not think the digestive system would have difficulty breaking down a meal with multiple kinds of foods in it. What is wrong with eating peanut butter and jelly sandwich with a cheesy bean and beef burrito and a fruit salad? It would seem harmless since Nature provides food in perfect packages combining fat, protein and sugar. If a kernel of corn is in a perfect blended ratio of protein, fat and carbohydrates, we should be able to eat a meal with these combinations as well, right? Well, yes and no.

Let's look at it this way. If you were a human animal, surviving off the land like your ancestors did, would it be possible to have an ancient buffet of buffalo steak and salmon, with corn on the cob, potato, spring snap peas, lentils, peanuts, cabbage and a dessert of bananas, apples, watermelon, pineapple and strawberries washed down with an eggnog? The answer is absolutely NOT! Unless your ancestor was from Krypton, had the name Superman and could leap from continent to continent in a single bound! It would be quite impossible to eat all these different types of food at one meal because they come from many different parts of the globe. What is more, these foods are harvested at different seasons. If you only lived on foods which were in season in your local area, you would not be able to eat all these foods at the same meal.

Four Seasons Dining

With modern methods of transporting food, it is possible for us to eat foods from different climates and in different seasons. This is not as Nature intended, and it may not be the healthiest option. Nature provides specific foods with the exact nutritional qualities needed by the beings living in that particular environment. In the warmer seasons of spring and summer and in warmer climates, Nature provides an abundance of food from plants, such as vegetables and fruits at the peak of their growing seasons.

Food from plants is lower in calories, easier on the digestion and provides less heat to the body. Less heat is needed to keep the body in a state of metabolic warmth because the ambient air temperature is higher. These plant-based foods are also loaded with colorful antioxidants which protect the plant from the harmful rays of the sun. When they are eaten by humans or animals, they in turn protect their cells from the intense summer sun. Spring and summer is also when Nature provides the lighter animal proteins like fresh fish and newly laid eggs from fowl.

During the fall and winter however, the foods which are more readily available are the root vegetables such as carrots, beets, parsnips and turnips. The winter apples, squashes, cabbages and cruciferous vegetables like broccoli, Brussels sprouts, collards, and kale are in season. Dried beans, nuts and seeds, as well as animal protein from wild game and fowl are all plentiful. These foods are all richer in energy and burn hotter to provide more energy in cooler climates and cold seasonal temperatures. If you eat too much of the rich, cold-weather foods like meat, fat and complex carbohydrates during the hot summer climate, you may find it difficult to shed the pounds. On the other hand, eating only greens and veggies and fruit during the winter may make you feel cold, hungry and fatigued because the body needs more energy and warmth.

Mixing and Matching

One of the big no-nos in food combination is the pairing of a meat or other heavy protein with a fruit. Fruits in general need little energy to be digested. They move through the digestive track relatively quickly. If fruit, which is digested quickly, is combined with a heavy meat, which requires longer digestion, what ensues is a gas bomb ready to erupt. The meat is not held in the gut long enough because the sugars and acids from the fruit are sending messages to the brain saying, "Come on, move me out!" At the same time, the fruit is being held too long because the meat protein and fat are sending messages to the brain saying, "Keep me in the stomach longer because I am not digested yet!" The result is a fermented mess.

These problems are compounded further if you eat a wide variety of processed foods all at the same meal. Do you remember the feeling in your gut after chowing down at an all-you-can-eat smorgasbord? Iceberg lettuce salad, bean salad, potato salad, and don't forget the fruit salad and those "Jello™-blended surprise" salads. Mix that mess together with reconstituted artificial mashed potatoes drowned in artificially-flavored gravy, creamed corn, macaroni and cheese, roast beef, ham, and spicy chicken legs. Then wash it down with soda pop and top it all off with chocolate cake and an ice cream sundae at the end! Yikes! It doesn't take much of a scientist to realize that eating a combination like this is going to cause some disturbance. In our family it was a disturbance which resulted in the car windows' being rolled down on the drive home! And it wasn't because we liked fresh air! ☺

One ancient therapy used for healing digestive complaints and other chronic illness was placing the patient on a "mono-diet." At each meal, the patient was given only one kind of food. This may have been a bowl of rice, a piece of fish, a potato, or a single type of other vegetable. The reason was to minimize the digestive stress on someone who wasn't well. The leftover energy conserved by not having to process heavy meals could be used instead to heal the body. This inherently makes sense; if you are spending too much energy processing and breaking down food, how much energy will be left for the detoxification of the body? What energy will be left over for the production of hormones or for the strengthening the immune system?

Because a mono-diet is quite difficult for the average person to maintain, I suggest to patients that they modify this principle to gain the benefits of a simplified diet but which will also provide the variety the taste buds crave. In order to maintain this balance it is necessary to limit the number of each different type of food eaten at each meal. For example, choose one type of protein (eggs, fish, chicken, beef, etc.) and one type of starch (potato, corn, rice, bread, etc.). Vegetables can be more generously included because they have similar rates of digestion and when mixed with the starch and protein the fiber from the vegetables actually helps to prevent food from being absorbed too quickly. Remember from Day 5, this is a great trick for keeping weight in a balanced level. Fats, oils, nuts and seeds can also be mixed with any types of food.

Eat it Alone

Fruit on the other hand, is never eaten with the meal because of its fast digestion. As my mentor once told me, "Eat it alone or leave it alone!" Choose to eat fruit as it was suggested in Day 6 and eat it no less than 30 minutes before a meal or wait until an hour after a meal. Fruit should not be mixed with other fruit which is either not in season or is from different climates. Don't mix apples with citrus, pineapples with berries, or bananas with plums. Mix only fruits which are compatible with those found growing in the same climatic location. Interestingly, fruits seem to combine well mixed with fats. An example would be fruit in combination with raw nuts and seeds or nut butter. The extra fat mixes well with the fruit and slows the absorption of the sugars into the bloodstream.

If fruit is cooked, such as in applesauce or preserves, then it is allowable for the fruit to be mixed with other foods in the place of the starch. Applesauce can be a healthy carbohydrate in place of potatoes, for example. The heat breaks down proteins and enzymes in the fruit which may cause allergic reactions in some people and it also breaks down fruit fibers and acids making it more digestible. People who can't tolerate raw fruit can usually eat it cooked. Adding half a ripe banana to oatmeal while it is cooking is a warm and delicious combination that does not create the gas that raw bananas sometimes can.

You may have heard that humans should not eat a protein and a starch at the same meal, such as meat and bread. If meat is digested primarily by the acidity in the stomach and bread digested primarily by the alkaline pancreatic enzymes, it would make sense not to eat these at the same time so as not to neutralize the digestion. If you eat the bread first, which is commonly done at a restaurant, the stomach acid gets soaked up by the bread. When you swallow the meat later in the meal, the stomach acids needed to break down the meat are now not as concentrated because they were absorbed by the bread. So, eat the meat first, the vegetables second and the starch last and eat them all slowly. Make sure to chew completely and mix the food with the saliva well to begin the first stage of digestion.

As mentioned earlier, food made by Nature is often packaged to combine protein, starch and fats so our digestive systems must have been intended to handle this combination. In general, it should not be an issue for most people with good digestion and no physical ailments. On the other hand, those with weaker digestion should be more aware of how they are combining the starches and proteins they are eating. In people with weak digestion, carbohydrates should be combined with vegetables and protein should be combined with vegetables. If you have multiple digestive issues, the simpler your food choices are, the better. Again, a mono-diet has been shown to be quite beneficial for people with digestive complaints but it is not an easy solution for many people.

Rotate Round and Round

While on the topic of food combinations, let us also briefly look at the importance of having a varied diet through the rotation of foods. In Nature, animals are not able to eat the same foods every day through the entire year because the seasons change and with it so does the climate. This means their diet changes accordingly. Likewise, if you get too comfortable with a particular menu, not only will it soon become boring, but it could also lead to health imbalances.

First, when you don't eat a variety of foods you don't get the variety of nutrition needed by the body. Some foods are higher in proteins, others in fats or carbohydrates, still others in minerals and vitamins. In order to receive a wide variety of nutrients from your foods, you have to make sure your food is rotated or kept varied.

And, some people have predispositions to food allergies. Their immune systems are actually fighting the food they are consuming for their sustenance. Not a good thing. We want the immune system to be fighting off bacteria, viruses, molds, fungus and parasites. It should not be spending time reacting to the food we are ingesting.

There are several classes of allergic responses. One type is called fast allergic reactions or anaphylactic allergies. These are the dangerous allergies in which the immune system responds with IgE antibodies. This is the type of allergy in which someone needs to be rushed to the hospital because his or her throat is closing. This is not the type of allergic response I am referring to here. Rather, what I find more pertinent when discussing food allergies are the insidious "slow response allergies" from IgA and IgG immunoglobulins.

These are called slow-response allergies because the reaction occurs over days instead of immediately. They can be associated with low-grade, long-term, chronic symptoms. I have been hugely impressed to see children with chronic ear, sinus or throat infections, enlarged tonsils, swollen eyes, plugged noses, behavioral and sleep disorders, skin reactions and asthma have their symptoms improve by eliminating these slow allergens. These slow allergies are commonly initiated by eating foods that Nature never intended for us to eat anyway (like processed foods and milk products). They are exacerbated by eating these same foods repeatedly. See a holistic physician if you are interested in having food allergies checked for IgG or IgA immunoglobulins or see Sources in back of this book for companies which run the necessary tests.

You can minimize slow IgG and IgA allergic responses and nutritional deficiencies by rotating and varying your food. This is especially beneficial with foods that tend to be allergenic, such as dairy products, wheat products, eggs, soy, citrus fruits and peanuts. I refer to it as the three-day rule; every three days make sure the food is rotated. This can be accomplished in one of two ways.

One method of rotating your food is to eat one type of food every few days. For example, if you have eggs on Monday, don't eat them again until Thursday. In the other method, you can eat the same food for three consecutive days, then switch and choose other types of food for the next week before returning to the first food. So, you can have peanut butter on toast for three days running for breakfast and then take a break and return to it a week later. Either of these approaches will bring variety in the form of nutrition and also lessen the possibility of aggravating subtle food allergies.

START TODAY:

- So for today use food-combining principles and keep your food choices as simple as possible. Choose one type of protein, one type of starch and a huge serving of vegetables preferably raw at each meal.

- Eat no fruit with the meal. Eat fruit only 30 minutes before or an hour after. Fruits are to be eaten alone and in their own seasonal and climate group and mixed only with nuts or fat.

- Rotate the foods from here on out by following the 3 day rule. See the back of the book for menu plans and see Nature's Diet Cookbook for recipe ideas.

Summary: This is what I'm doing up to this point, each day adds onto the next

Day 1: Food awareness: Keep a diary of my foods. I am accountable.

Day 2: Water: Sip half my body weight in ounces throughout the day.

Day 3: Movement: Some exercise performed every day. Note it in my diary.

Day 4: Regular meals: Eat about the same time each day.

Day 5: Vegetables and Raw Living Foods: 50% of total weight of your food.

Day 6: Fruit: Up to 2 servings of locally grown fruit daily (no fruit juice)

Day 7: Carbohydrates: One serving per meal combined with vegetables.

Day 8: Protein: One serving of healthy animal protein at every meal.

Day 9: FAT: Eliminate bad fats and add one serving of good fat per meal.

Day 10: Grocery shopping, food preparation, condiments, and serving sizes.

Day 11: Practical food combining: Mix, match, and rotate properly.

Day 12
Breakfast

It took us a while to work up to this one and in a moment you will see why. Of course, you've have heard that breakfast is the most important meal of the day and that is the truth. "Breaking the fast" properly from the night's sleep is an important step in boosting your wellness. Traditionally, our breakfasts in the Western world are excessively loaded with foods high in sugar and rich in grease. We love our breakfast cereals, pastries and donuts, jam and toast, glasses of fruit juice. We also love those greasy artificially flavored processed foods like sausage, bacon, ham, and fake cheeses.

Just looking at the typical morning breakfast plate, it would be hard to identify where any of the foods came from in Nature. Most foods bear no resemblance at all to the foods they used to be prior to processing and preparation. This is a good way to determine which foods are healthful and which most likely are not. If the food item still looks like the original whole food as found in Nature, then it is probably okay. Maple bars, Fruit Loops™, pancakes with syrup, wiener links, and cheese omelets look nothing like the natural foods from which they were originally made.

If you were from another planet and never saw earth food before, could you tell what plant or animal in Nature these foods came from just by looking at them? Obviously not! These foods are so heavily processed and manipulated by humans that it no longer possible to identify where in Nature they came from. Our food has been highly processed and altered to satisfy our demands for flavor, fast preparation, extended shelf-life, and of course, our tight budgets.

Our ancestors never had access to pre-packaged breakfast cereals, deep fried hash browns, pop tarts, lattés, or even orange juice! They ate what Nature provided for them. These foods were already prepared by Nature as being ready to eat in their own perfect packages, not adulterated with salt, sugar, artificial flavors or colors. Remember too, the processing of foods and the addition of chemicals as flavor-enhancers and preservatives have only been around for a couple hundred years. Our human genes have been around for many hundreds of thousands of years, constantly adapting to our environment. Our genes have not had sufficient time to adapt to the artificial man-made chemicals found in breakfast foods such as Lucky Charms™, Kraft Singles™, and Jimmy Dean's™ sausages which have only been available for the past few decades.

Arise and Shine

Changing the first meal of the day can do much to improve the health of people on this planet. Starting the day off with the traditional highly concentrated sugary and greasy breakfasts causes the pancreas to over-secrete insulin. This is no problem if it happens occasionally, but when insulin is secreted like this meal after meal, the body becomes insensitive to these high levels, resulting eventually in obesity and type-2 diabetes. This is a growing epidemic in our country, especially among children. Breakfast cereals with incredibly high levels of sugar and artificial ingredients are one of the worst health atrocities of our time. We are feeding our children a breakfast which causes their pancreas to start the day with an insulin surge. The body works desperately to recuperate from these highs and lows for the remainder of the day. Our children are becoming fatter and fatter and it isn't by chance.

This is a good time to talk about energy bars and protein shakes. Neither of these artificial foods are excuses for meals! They are quite unnatural and often consist of concentrated ingredients which are highly processed. Many of these bars are high in sugars and combined with a processed soy or whey powder which is a milk product. Protein in this powdered and processed form is NOT NATURAL and not as usable by the body as protein which comes directly from real food.

Proteins are best eaten as Nature intended - in their whole meat, egg, nut, or seed forms. Consider drinking raw egg smoothies blended with rice milk and almond butter in place of these artificially processed protein shakes. Eggs and nut or seed butters combine to make an excellent source of whole natural protein and fat. Raw nuts and seeds make great snacks in place of energy bars. Be careful with dried fruits like raisins, craisins, figs, and prunes as well because they contain a high concentration of sugar. Eating them in small amounts mixed with raw nuts and seeds like a trail mix will slow the absorption of too much sugar into the body at once. You may also choose to sweeten grains or cooked breakfast cereals by rehydrating the dried fruit in the water while the grain is cooking.

Dinner at Breakfast

So how is the best way to start the day? Well, we want to start the day eating like our ancestors did thousands of years ago and many cultures still do today. If you travel around the world you will observe that many countries (particularly developing countries) traditionally do not eat the same types of foods for breakfasts that Westerners do. They start the day with a hearty or bland meal as opposed to sugary, sweet and greasy breakfasts. Such healthy breakfasts include beans and rice south of the border, soup and rice in Asia, or yams and stew in Africa. These options are a big difference from the intensified carbohydrate load of the West.

Since you are almost at the end of your second week, it is time to really step up this program and become even braver. So I am going to encourage you to do what I ask of all my patients; to try to imitate what is done all around the world for the first meal. Instead of sugary sweet, you are going to start the day off with lunch or dinner types of food for breakfast. Yes! It is really very simple too. Just prepare enough food from dinner the night before so you have leftovers for breakfast the next morning. As strange as it sounds to have chicken soup or beans and avocado or steak fajitas or even a sandwich and salad for breakfast, that is what your goal will be.

Dinner and lunch foods are high in good quality protein, fats, minerals and essential nutrients like minerals, vitamins and essential fatty acids. They are also much lower in sugary sweetness than traditional breakfasts. By starting the day with a more balanced meal you will not suffer that mid-morning sugar drop which results in fatigue and sleepiness. People who eat foods lower in sugar invariably have more balanced weight and mood than those eating traditional American breakfasts. With this change you will boost your nutrition and thus your overall health.

For some of you, the very thought of this may be turning your stomach as you read. For you folks, instead of jumping right into liver and onions with spinach salad for breakfast, start with something you can manage, such as eggs and toast or eggs and whole grain cereal. When you get brave try starting the day with soup; try any type from chicken vegetable soup to lentil soup. Eventually, the transition to really brave choices such as chicken stir-fry or fish with steamed veggies and brown rice. Maybe, just maybe, you will eventually be able to wake up to a nice cut of sautéed liver and onions on a bed of spinach!

Some people have difficulty eating anything until lunch. In this case a small serving of locally grown seasonal fruit can be a good option for those who need something light with which to start the day. However, it is inadequate for a complete breakfast and it absolutely must be followed by a complete breakfast an hour later. The small serving of fruit only allows the digestive system to be gently awakened after the night's rest.

In the back of this book you'll find meal ideas to help create a menu plan that will work for you. The items are not listed as breakfast, lunch or dinner because these foods are balanced for any meal any time of the day. You no longer need to be concerned about breakfast foods for breakfast or dinner foods for dinner, so long as you have the proper balance of nutrition to bring health as Nature intended. Wake up tomorrow and pull out the soup or sandwich or the roasted chicken and rice and veggies and see how different your morning and day become!

START TODAY:

- Choose a non-sweet, non-traditional breakfast. If you are brave go for a full-on dinner or lunch for breakfast. If you need some encouragement, start with eggs and toast or eggs and whole grain cereal.

- No protein bars or protein shake powders allowed. Try the eggnog suggestion under the meal planner options in the back of the book. A list of snack recommendations is listed with the menu options.

Summary: This is what I'm doing up to this point, each day adds onto the next

Day 1: **Food awareness:** Keep a diary of my foods. I am accountable.

Day 2: **Water:** Sip half my body weight in ounces throughout the day.

Day 3: **Movement:** Some exercise performed every day. Note it in my diary.

Day 4: **Regular meals:** Eat about the same time each day.

Day 5: **Vegetables and Raw Living Foods:** 50% of total weight of your food.

Day 6: **Fruit:** Up to 2 servings of locally grown fruit daily (no fruit juice).

Day 7: **Carbohydrates:** One serving per meal combined with vegetables.

Day 8: **Protein:** One serving of healthy animal protein at every meal.

Day 9: **FAT:** Eliminate bad fats and add one serving of good fat per meal.

Day 10: Grocery shopping, food preparation, condiments, and serving sizes.

Day 11: Practical food combining: Mix, match, and rotate properly.

Day 12: Dinner or lunch type meals for breakfast (MENU IN THE BACK).

Day 13
Artificial Chemicals, Drugs, & Toxic Pollution

B y now, I hope you are beginning to understand the concept of the Healing Power of Nature. You can have optimal physical and emotional health by observing Nature and following the natural laws of science. The first medical doctor, Hippocrates, felt the role of the doctor was to provide the body with what was needed and to remove the obstacles which prevented the body from healing itself. So far, we have been talking about providing the body with what it needs in the form of the nutrition for repair and regeneration. Now we will discuss the obstacles that must be removed in order for the healing to take place.

The greatest obstacles to cure are man-made chemicals. These chemicals are artificial substances not found anywhere in Nature. They come to us in our processed foods, our medicines, our household chemicals, and in our environmental pollution. Less than two hundred years ago, mankind's diet consisted completely of food which was hunted from the land, harvested from their own garden, or raised by a local farmer. Today, we sustain ourselves almost entirely with foods which are processed or already prepared ready-to-eat from boxes, cans, packages or restaurants.

Even sugar, which at one time was considered a prized commodity eaten only on special occasions, is now eaten in excessive amounts from the time we are able to eat until we die. Today the average consumption of sugar and other sweeteners per American per year is 140 pounds! In other words, some people are eating more sugar than the weight of their own bodies! Compare that to the sugar consumption of one hundred years ago - only 5 pounds per person per year. Can you see how conditions caused by excess sugar consumption such as obesity, diabetes, high cholesterol and triglycerides, and heart disease are major epidemics?

Sugar is a perfect example of a food which started as a healthful natural food before it was transformed by man into a substance which acts more like a drug. The sugar you buy in the store never looked like white crystal power when it was harvested from Nature. It began as a crispy dark green plant that looks like a big, tall stalk of grass. This green stalk was cut and the juice was pressed to make a refreshing, sweet, greenish-brown liquid which was delicious and nutritious.

This liquid was then dehydrated to make very concentrated dark brown crystal granules much sweeter than the liquid but still loaded with B vitamins and minerals. Finally, these brown granules were further processed and refined. The nutrients were washed away and the brown color was bleached with chemicals to make a very, very concentrated sweetener. The final product is that white, sweet powdery stuff that you purchase from the store called "SUGAR". The final product has no resemblance to the plant that Nature gave us.

Feel Good Flavors

With scientific progress and technological advancement, industry's ability to create artificial flavors and food enhancers has become a huge and massively profitable industry. Artificial flavors and chemical enhancers are designed as less expensive substitutes for more costly natural flavors. They save money and they enhance the flavors of food so not only is it cheaper but it is tastier and that means we are going to be attracted to it. Tastier food stimulates neurological pathways in the brain so that we crave these foods. This is literally the beginning of an addiction.

When these rich, artificially flavored foods are eaten daily, the taste buds are conditioned to want only foods with tons of flavor. When this happens, wholesome natural food seems bland and less attractive. The brain craves, or is actually "addicted" to, foods which are artificially processed and made with chemical flavor enhancers. Our taste buds have become acclimated to the adulterated food.

These flavor enhancers are even finding their way into pet food. Have you ever given your puppy or kitty a serving of canned pet food and watched their reaction? If they are like most animals, they will eat their dry food or enjoy a table scrap now and again. This prepared food from a can is like a crack addiction to them. They slurp it down so fast and then come running back for more. They would eat the whole thing at once if they could and of course that means you have to buy more. The manufacturers know this and they are doing it to *your* food as well.

So if artificial flavor enhancers are stimulating our taste buds, what does this really mean? It means our taste buds have been set to a higher level of stimulation. Therefore, we feel satisfied only when we eat these rich artificial foods. Consequently, we will only be attracted to these artificially enhanced foods and our desire for whole natural foods will diminish. In short: WE ARE ADDICTED TO THESE FLAVOR-ENHANCED FOODS. Literally, we are now ADDICTED to a new flavor of food because the REAL FOOD DOESN'T TASTE GOOD ANYMORE. That means big money for the manufacturer because you just keep coming back for more! Like we really needed one more addiction right? It really is all about the money.

Drugged by Dopamine

How do these chemicals affect the brain? They stimulate the release of dopamine in the brain which makes us want to go back for more. Whether the person is addicted to drugs, alcohol or fast food, dopamine is released in the brain causing the addiction. Dopamine is the "feel good" molecule; it elevates both emotional and physical feelings of elation. These chemicals are usually added to foods that are the worst for our waistline because they are loaded with fat, sugar, salt and empty calories. So, we get fatter and fatter; we can't stay on a diet because nothing tastes good, and we wonder why we just keep going back to that bag of Doritos™. For some reason no matter how hard we try we can't eat just one! (They were right! What did they know that we didn't?)

These artificial chemical enhancers are added to most processed and prepared foods, especially food that is convenient for us to open the package and pop it right into our mouths! Quick, fast, and easy! That's what processed food is about, the ease of convenience and preparation. Whether it is a frozen pizza or lasagna, that Hungry Man™ TV dinner, the breakfast cereal from a box, most food from restaurants especially fast food, snacks such as chips, cookies, candies and drinks such as sodas, juices and sport drinks, they are all considered processed food. Even though the ingredients from which they were made, originally started out as a healthy whole food grown or raised on a farm.

At one time, the ingredients could have been identified as grains, vegetables and meats harvested from Nature. Now they are refined, processed and given flavors which have been chemically enhanced. They have been treated with colors and preservatives to give them better visual appearance and a long shelf-life. The end result is a food which, when compared to food found in Nature, looks better, feels better in your mouth, and of course tastes so much better... it is OUT OF THIS WORLD! And it is true! It is not found anywhere in this natural world!!!

A Junk Food Junkie Is Rehabilitated

The following is a letter from a 25 year old female patient of mine who wrote me after making a series of changes to her diet.

Dear Dr. Iverson,

I wanted to share with you what has happened to me since I have taken your suggestions and changed my diet. As you know, I have lived the majority of my life eating very unhealthy and unnatural foods. Ever since I could eat solid foods, I have eaten fast food an average of four times a week. If it wasn't fast food, then my parents prepared me meals that were frozen or from a box or a can. In between meals, I snacked on candy, chips, cookies, soda pop, and junk food of any kind.

I feel fortunate to have good genes, so I have never been overweight despite my poor eating habits. However, after my medical visit with you, I realized that I may be causing harm that I wasn't able to see such as the breakdown of my teeth and bones. After hearing that I wasn't as healthy as I thought I was, I decided to take your advice and follow your diet plan. This included drinking water in place of soda and replacing whole foods in place of fast food and processed food.

I knew that changing my diet would be difficult for someone like me. My taste buds desired foods that were highly flavored. All I wanted to eat was fast food. I was simply addicted to it. The thought of vegetables without ranch dressing or cheese sauce and fruits without whipping cream or chocolate syrup repulsed me. I had never eaten anything labeled "natural" or "organic" in my life. Nevertheless, I began the dietary changes as you instructed.

The first two days were hard. The next three were worse. After a full plate of vegetables, lean meat, and whole grain rice (which I could barely stand eating), I still was not satisfied. My mind turned this dissatisfaction into a feeling of hunger. I was hungry for grease, sugar, salt, carbohydrates, and food with flavor...artificial flavor that is. The cravings were so strong that I became irritable. I was salivating at every restaurant commercial on television and arguing with myself why I was doing this. Since it was too soon to notice any results, I felt unhappy and bewildered and I felt like I was treating myself unfairly.

A week passed by and it was then that I began to notice some amazing changes in my body. My entire life I have been constipated having just one bowel movement every 3-4 days. Within one week I became regular having daily bowel movements. Besides this I noticed I did not have heartburn after eating anymore.

This was enough of a change that I really started paying attention to the other possible signs of healing. People at work started to tell me that my body looked tone and my skin was clearer than they ever remember. I was in a better mood too. I'm not sure if that was because I was receiving so many compliments or I was having better brain chemistry.

And then, something amazing happened in my life. Since I

was a little girl in elementary school I had difficulty waking up in the morning. Regardless of how much sleep I had the night before it was nearly impossible for me to wake up. I would hit the snooze on my alarm over and over without knowing it. I tried everything to correct this problem but nothing worked. As a result, I struggled in school and later I had even lost jobs because of this.

After just a week now, I am shocked at how my body is responding. Now, I am waking up every morning before my alarm clock sounds. Amazingly I am even doing this if I only had five hours of sleep the night before. To think that at one time I was seriously considering seeing a therapist because I thought I must be depressed. Just by improving my diet, I realized that I was not depressed at all. I was poisoning myself with processed food!

Every new day I feel I am becoming stronger and healthier. I am sleeping more soundly and I recall my dreams more often than I ever have. I have energy that lasts throughout the whole day. My mind is clear and focused and I am motivated to complete my next project. And can you believe it, I no longer have a craving for my favorite fast food burger anymore?

Recently I was at work and one of my co-workers was on a lunch break. I watched her eat her Crunchwrap Supreme from Taco Bell. That used to be my favorite item on the menu. What actually caught my attention was the way she was eating it. She was taking every bite and chewing it as if she was in ecstasy. She was "mmmmming" and "ahhhhhing" and saying aloud how delicious it was. What a sight. It was then I realized that girl was me at one time. I wasn't able to see my addiction until I was able to eliminate fast food and processed food from my life.

I just can't believe I have dealt with these symptoms for so many years and the doctors had no answer for a kid that was tired all day and couldn't get out of bed. I just can't believe it was really as easy as changing my diet to Nature's foods. My life is so different now and it makes me happier than words can explain. I can't thank you enough. Please share this so others so they may also be helped.

Wow! What awesome testimony to the power of following Nature's Diet! To imagine that this young lady could have lived her entire life feeling that she was destined for fatigue and depression. Can you imagine what could have happened as her body aged and she didn't have the minerals to maintain strong bones and healthy cells? Is it any wonder our children who eat school lunches loaded with chemical additives along with fast food and junk food are having difficulty maintaining their grades? As you read, she even lost her job because she couldn't function! Is it any wonder why the U.S. is one of the unhealthiest countries in the world, with an epidemic of heart disease, diabetes and cancer? This patient's testimony can teach us much about the root causes of disease in our fast food nation.

Out of This World

It is important to understand that many of the chemicals in our food and environment are not found naturally on this planet. Our genes have not been exposed to them until recently in the long history of the human race. Our genes and our DNA, early in human existence, were exposed to Nature's own chemicals found in the soil, in plants and in other animals. Because of this long period of co-existence, our DNA has adapted to these naturally occurring chemicals over time.

Chemicals, as created by Man, have accompanied us into a new age of efficiency, making our lives much easier in many ways, but with a price. We are dependent on these chemicals to operate our cars, to add color to our lives with paints and dyes, to purify our water, to clean our toilets and clothes with detergents, and to clean our bodies with soaps, shampoos and toothpastes. And the list goes on. We are exposed to literally thousands of man-made chemicals every day, some much more toxic than others. That is an incredible load of chemicals that your miraculous and splendid liver and kidneys are forced to filter from your blood every day.

To all these chemicals to which we are exposed on a daily basis, we add even more via the most direct route: right into our mouths! Unlike the toxins in your environment, the chemicals in your food are something you can control and make a conscientious choice to avoid. If you can lower the chemical burden on your body in any way by choosing not to put them in your body, you will be taking a vital step to promoting better health.

Unlike the chemicals Nature herself created, man-made chemicals are so new, relative to the entire time of human existence, that our DNA has not yet adapted to the harmful effects they can have. An estimated 75,000 different chemicals are used in the U.S. alone![1] The vast majority of these chemicals are completely unregulated by governing bodies because their long-term effects are largely unknown. It is estimated that our population as a whole carries trace amounts of several hundred different chemicals. In your body alone it is estimated that you are carrying an average of 56 chemicals which have been linked to cancer, heart disease, nervous system degenerative diseases, hormone alterations, reproductive inhibition and birth defects.[2] With so many different kinds of foreign chemicals to clear from the blood, it is evident that the body could get over-burdened and the immune system confused, resulting in the rise of numerous diseases that were once rare or unknown.

Entire books have been written about the effects of chemicals on our environment and on the human body; it is not within the scope of this book to cover them in detail. You might recognize some of their names as listed in a table at the end of this chapter. It is fair to say, though, that major diseases are on the rise. It is especially alarming to see increases in illnesses which have been associated with toxic chemicals and heavy metal exposure. Cancer, autoimmune disorders, cardiovascular events, hormonal disorders leading to infertility, and neurological diseases all have been connected to increased exposure to chemical toxins.

Medication Madness

Even though modern medicine has come far in its technological advances and will continue to do so in the future, it is important to realize that prescription drug medications are also man-made chemicals not found anywhere in Nature. According to studies, it is estimated that 100,000 people die from medications which are properly administered, making it the 4th leading cause of death in America![3] That follows closely behind heart disease, cancer and stroke, as the top four big killers. Among these four it is the most easily controlled because medications are chemicals we choose to ingest. And to think that these are deaths due to prescription medications which are properly administered by a doctor! This number does not include people who have overdosed from prescription medications like pain killers. These are quickly becoming the most abused "recreational" substances.

Again, our genes have not had the time to adapt to these foreign chemical medications. When these chemicals interact with the millions of other chemical naturally occurring in your body it can make for a deadly cocktail. Medications can be life-saving, but they can also be life-taking so they must be used judiciously. The future of responsible medicine lies in blending the best of modern scientific technology with the wisdom of Nature's principles for living well. Thomas Edison saw the early dangers of chemical drugs prescribed for illness as he wrote this statement, *"The doctor of the future will give no medicine, but will interest his patients in the care of the human body, in diet, and in the cause and prevention of disease."*

As an aside, the growing popularity of cholesterol medication is being hailed as the answer for a country which is reaping the negative effects of eating contrary to Nature. A person who consumes chemically-enhanced food for decades, water which is chemically altered, drinks which are loaded with artificial sweeteners, stimulating caffeine or nicotine is definitely going to show increases in cholesterol over time. Add this to the daily exposure of chemical toxins found in the home, workplace and environment and what do you get? A combination for INFLAMMATION!

Our bodies are screaming for help. They are hot and red and burning from this daily assault! In its great wisdom, the body manufactures little band-aids we call cholesterol to lie down on blood vessels and soothe the inflamed or injured tissue. Cholesterol is the body's natural response to our poor living in a very imperfect, industrialized, artificial world.

Of course, as far as we know, there is no tree or plant that bears the fruit of Lipitor™ or Zocor™ to take care of our elevated inflammation (C-reactive protein) and cholesterol levels! This is where the indiscriminate use of medications has become an absurd falsification. We think that we can continue to live the life we live, with all its pleasures of food and convenience, and by taking a drug all symptoms will just go away. Just take this for that or this for that. With one simple pill we can continue to eat our diets of decay, ignore the need for exercise, avoid the stress in our life, and still take years off. We simply want our cake and we want to eat it too! (We certainly are eating a lot of cake these days!)

Unfortunately, Nature never intended this. It is showing us that something is not right with our "logical" solution by virtue of our increasing health problems. It also begs the question: if these medications are so valuable as life-savers, why is the U.S. still considered one of the unhealthiest countries in the world? How do other countries continue to survive without these so called "life saving drugs?" I'm sure Haitians and Hondurans are not falling over from heart attacks because they lack Lipitor™. What about the lack of Prozac™ or Wellbutrin™ for people who live in Ethiopia or Bangladesh? Even though they have a lot more to be anxious or depressed about than we do (given their economic state), do they need to take medication to withstand their emotional hardships?

What does a third-world country have that we don't? Yeah, that is right, big business making tons of money from us wealthy folk with chemical foods and chemical medications. If we continue to pollute our bodies and our earth with these chemicals, the results will be more of the same. We will continue to become sicker and more tired and diseased, falling farther and farther from Nature's plan. Dr. Arden Anderson is a conventionally trained osteopathic doctor who wrote an informative book on natural healing titled, *Real Medicine Real Health*. These words from his book sum it up:

> *"The problem is that most doctors do not look at prescription medications as adjunct therapies to nutrition and diet. They look at prescription medications as first line therapy and diet and nutrition as no therapy at all."*
>
> Arden Anderson DO, PhD

Cure or Cover Up

While we are on the subject of medication and chemicals, it is important to understand that modern medicine is very limited in its ability to actually *cure* a disease. Yes, some surgeries may cure an incident, repairing a limb which was in a traumatic accident or a heart with a defective valve. The majority of treatments your doctor prescribes to you are merely palliative, which means it just relieves the symptoms as long as the treatment is being taken. When the treatment (drug) is discontinued, the symptom or the disorder returns. Inherently there is no cure because you, the patient, are dependent on the drug to keep the symptoms away. You have not been educated on how to treat the cause of the symptoms.

For example, even after a surgery which is successful in removing a tumor, the body's environment which potentially caused the tumor was never treated along with the tumor. The person whose genetics rendered them susceptible to tumors is still being exposed to the same toxic chemical environment that existed prior to the surgery. This means the condition will likely recur. In order to address the cause of the tumor's growth, the environment of the body must also be changed to prevent its happening again.

Drug medications are rarely curative. For example, a person who suffers with headaches every day takes pain relievers to make the pain go away. The pain goes away, but does it keep the headache from returning the next day? No, because the headache's cause is still there. The cause might be anything from a lack of minerals or imbalanced hormones, to poor sleep, but the medication did not provide a cure; it merely calmed or palliated the symptoms.

The drug companies know very well the difference between a palliation and an actual cure. Because sick people mean big business – and enormous profits – for drug companies, it is in their best interest for you to live out of alignment with Nature. Remember, if you are perfectly healthy and have no need for their drugs, the companies who make them would lose big money. Many drugs are taken for a lifetime; the intention is not to cure the illness. A real cure represents a recipe for self-destruction for any drug company.

One story I'll never forget was from a patient who came to see me for her elevated blood pressure and cholesterol. I explained that as her body becomes healthier through nutrition and lifestyle improvements, she may notice that her blood pressure and cholesterol will decrease on their own. I continued to explain that as values come into normal ranges we could expect to reduce or even eliminate the need for her two medications.

"What? Oh no, doctor! I couldn't possibly stop taking my medications! I need those medications so I don't have a heart attack," she said in a worried tone.

"Oh yes, for now you will need them until you get healthier, and then as your numbers drop you may not need them anymore," I reassured her.

"Oh no doctor, I can't ever stop taking my medications."

"Well if your blood pressure is optimal and your cholesterol levels are optimal without medication why would you need them? Did you need them when you were a young healthy girl?" I asked.

Regardless of my explanations of this principle, she was thoroughly convinced (brainwashed) that she could never forego that medication no matter how healthy she became.

Deadly Disease or Just a Deficiency?

You may currently have symptoms which are really just deficiencies currently being treated with drugs. Nutritional deficiencies from a diet poor in essential fatty acids, amino acids, vitamins, minerals and coenzymes can worsen over time and masquerade as a disease. If a person has the symptoms of a dry mouth, dizziness, changes in vision, headache and vomiting that person might think he or she needs pain medication or even an anti-nausea/vomiting medication. But what if the person said the symptoms started after hiking vigorously all day in the hot sun? In this case, drinking water would cure the symptoms which were actually caused by a lack of water. Can you see how we may have symptoms which are related to a deficiency but for which we take drugs to alleviate those symptoms instead of nourishing our body? Unfortunately, this is how we have been educated to care for ourselves when symptoms show up.

Many of our deficiency-related symptoms are self-induced and are created by our own choices. I like to use the example of an alcoholic hangover. You know why you are sick; it is because you drank too much alcohol the previous night. The alcohol drained your body of essential fluids and electrolytes and poisoned your liver. So you take aspirin or another pain reliever to calm the discomfort (which just adds more stress to the liver). Massive profits from pain medication sales have been enjoyed by the drug companies because of our occasional boozing it up. This is an example of a self-induced malady.

What about heartburn, indigestion, gas, belching and the ten million dollar word gastro-esophageal reflux disease or GERD? It too begins as a self-induced symptom caused by consistent poor food choices. It is not an illness that simply happened to you or because it just "runs in your family." It is something that inevitably happened to your body after years of abusing processed foods. Maybe eating unhealthy food "runs in your family" instead. Sooner or later your body will not recover from the chemical imbalance and either a hyper-acidic or hypo-acidic state will be created in your gut. The result of this is indigestion and heartburn. You may think the answer is a medication; the media, the drug companies and the drug-company-educated doctors all tell you this. So, believing these health authorities you buy Tums™, Prevacid™, Tagamet™, Prilosec™ or some other expensive (and profitable for the drug company) treatment.

Your immediate indigestion symptoms go away so you go about your own business eating the same junk food you always ate but now you pop a pill with it. This continues until new symptoms emerge and you receive a diagnosis of ulcers, gastritis, irritable bowel syndrome, diverticulitis or, God-forbid, cancer. Not to mention possible side effects such as bone loss. "But, why? I did what the doctors told me." Because you continued to feed your body the same chemical foods that caused the problem initially. You did not take good care of your body by changing your food choices. You continued to ignore the most benign warning signs your body was giving you. The indigestion was not a sign of a disease, it was a warning sign from the body to shape yourself up or ship yourself out!

Therefore, I teach my patients to be aware of how their bodies are talking to them. There are many so-called "illnesses" which are not actual diseases at all but just warning signs. Your body is waving flags and flashing messages, trying to make you wake up and change your life. You don't need more medication; you need to pay attention to your body. You need to pay attention to these mild symptoms now before it is too late; before you really do have a serious disease.

These are examples of symptoms which are early warning signs from your body. These are a call for help from your body asking you to change your life. Do you have headaches, muscle aches, joint pain, indigestion, constipation, diarrhea, blood sugar fluctuations, blood pressure elevations, cholesterol elevations, skin rashes, persistent colds and allergies, painful and heavy menstrual cycles, fatigue and sleeplessness, depressed or anxious moods, addictions, weight gain or loss? Have you taken a medication for any of these symptoms thinking it was a drug to cure your illness? Think again. Your body is telling you something. Pay attention to its whispers before they become roars. Change your life and change your lifestyle to promote better health.

Brain Excitement

Let's move on. What about your daily life? How can you control the foods you are consuming daily to make sure that you are choosing those foods which are less processed, which contain fewer man-made chemicals and which are more closely aligned with Nature?

Simply enough - you need to read labels! There is a lot to be said about a label which is lengthy and contains multiple words that are either unpronounceable or simply sound nasty. Some of these substances which find their way into our daily food supply can have serious implications for health, especially in people with neurological disorders like faulty attention span, and mood and pain conditions. Foods which have ingredients like monosodium glutamate (MSG), a flavor enhancer, and aspartame, which is an artificial sweetener found in products like Equal™, NutraSweet™, and Canderel™ can overly excite the nerve messages in the brain. Other hidden names for MSG are also yeast extract, autolyzed yeast extract, hydrolyzed vegetable protein, textured protein, sodium and calcium caseinate. Read your labels and compare to the table at the end of the chapter.

The brain uses two chemicals, glutamate and aspartate, as messengers to send nerve signals. When chemically enhanced foods with monosodium glutamate or aspartame are ingested, the naturally occurring chemicals in the brain can come out of balance. These chemicals are called "excito-toxins" because they have a stimulating or excitatory impact on the nervous system. This can cause some people to experience neurological symptoms affecting their behavior, their moods, and their pain levels.

Headaches, tingling and numbness, muscle or joint pain, attention disorders and hyperactivity disorders are a few of the most common conditions caused by these chemicals. Eliminating MSG, aspartame, artificial flavors, and artificial colors such as food dyes

(FD & C yellow and reds and blues etc) have been beneficial in helping people who have focus and behavioral disorders. In fact, many neurological disorders such as headaches, chronic pain, and mood changes like anxiety and depression have been associated with consuming these chemicals.

If your child is having trouble in school then maybe you should reassess his or her diet. If the child is fatigued or falling asleep in class, hard to wake in the morning, having difficulty listening or focusing on the assignments, or acting out or misbehaving, you may be seeing the effect of excito-toxins. Clean up the child's diet as recommended. Do not allow your child to eat fast food and do not allow permit school lunches which are usually loaded with chemical enhancers and fillers. Prepare all meals at home, being cautious to read all labels and avoid the chemicals in the list below.

Sweet Surrender

Even more simply, start first by eliminating that most basic of processed foods: WHITES! White foods are usually refined foods. They are foods which were originally harvested from Nature in a more complete and wholesome form. For example, white rice was actually brown rice before its brown hull covering was polished away from it; the brown hull which was discarded contains very high levels of nutrients. In order to obtain more nutrition from your food, you need to exchange processed white foods for the healthier versions that Nature originally provided.

Instead of white bread, choose the whole grain sprouted bread. White bread is made from whole wheat which has been stripped of the hull and bleached; yes, bleached with chemicals! Does that sound like a "Wonder" to you? Instead of white rice choose brown or wild rice; instead of large white potatoes choose baby reds or yellow or yams or sweet potatoes. Instead of white pasta choose whole-grain or vegetable pastas. Remember, the more refined and purified the food is, the less nutrition is left in it. This is why even the bread purchased as "whole wheat" will say "enriched flour." It is really just white wheat flour with some whole-wheat flour mixed in and some vitamins added because the nutrients had already stripped away. Whole wheat bread is really just processed white bread hiding undercover; read the labels.

It is very important to avoid food which has high fructose corn syrup as one of its ingredients. It is a CHEMICALLY MADE, FAKE SUGAR, just like the other fake sweeteners Nutrasweet™, Equal™ and Splenda™. These are difficult for the body to metabolize. Candies, pastries, soda pop and sport drinks are some of the highest sources of high fructose corn syrup. Remember, one 8 ounce cup of Coke™ has 26 grams of sugar. That is more than 6 teaspoons!

Fructose is not a health food. When kept in its natural form as found in Nature, the small amount of fructose found in fruit is not serious. This fructose is combined with natural plant fibers so it is more dilute. However, when it is processed and concentrated as a sweetener, it is toxic. Fructose is a sugar which is metabolized directly by the liver and is even more lipogenic or fat-inducing than glucose. This means the fructose promotes the making and storing of fat in your body especially the liver.

As fat levels rise, not only do we get a fatty body but we also get a fatty liver. A fatty liver can cause insulin resistance, elevated triglycerides, and increased "bad" LDL cholesterol as well as increased uric acid and lactic acid levels. The result is an increase in obesity, diabetes, heart disease, fatty liver disease, kidney stones, and gout.[4] It is no surprise that we are becoming overweight as we substitute soda and sport drinks for water!

If "sugar" is written on the ingredient label, it is more than likely refined white sugar as described earlier. A good alternative is to select foods with natural sugars as found in Nature, such as raw honey, grade B pure maple syrup (grade A is too refined), beet sugar, molasses, and Rapadura or Sucanat which is dehydrated sugar cane juice. Even though these are still sugars and can still be damaging when take in excess, they are not nearly as processed as bleached white sugar.

Raw honey is Nature's most naturally concentrated sweetener, but it is not to be treated like a health food. It is the essence of nectar from flowers, concentrated by bees and insects. It consists of approximately 50% glucose and 50% fructose. Because it is 50% glucose, it can be put under the tongue for someone having a low blood sugar response to bring them out of it quickly. But, honey has as much fructose as high fructose corn syrup or white sugar. BE CAREFUL! In small amounts it can be enjoyed as a treat, but in excess it is every bit as harmful as all concentrated sugars in that it raises blood sugar, triglycerides and bad cholesterol and puts you at risk for diabetes and heart disease. Honey is a SURVIVAL FOOD for BEES over the wintertime, not for HUMANS. It is not meant to be eaten in large quantities.

A sweet tooth once in a while isn't going to destroy your health. If you want do still enjoy your treats, make them occasional (a couple times a week) instead of frequent. You want to allow enough time for the body to recuperate and detoxify from any harmful chemical byproducts. We'll talk more about sweets and treats soon.

Sweet Stand-off

For diabetics and people who are trying to avoid sugar, the natural sweeteners stevia, xylitol, and erythritol do not cause the same glucose-insulin responses regular sweeteners do. Even fructose from fruit is not good for diabetics because it can create the same diabetic diseases as too much glucose. What's worse, fructose levels cannot be monitored on a glucose meter because these are two different molecular compounds.

When you consume fructose, although your blood sugar doesn't rise as much as it does with sucrose, it still fills the blood with the simple sugar molecules. This is known as glycation and it still forms the same advanced glycation end products (AGEs) which can damage the eyes, kidneys and nerves of diabetics as glucose.[5] Diabetics do NOT want to use the artificial sweeteners aspartame, saccharin, sucralose or Splenda™ ever. These are all artificial substances that the body cannot recognize because THEY ARE NOT FOUND IN NATURE and their long-term effects are still unknown.

Stevia is a natural sweetener from the plant *Stevia rebaudiana*. It is originally from Paraguay and is much sweeter than sugar, but since it is not made from sugar it does not raise glucose levels in the blood. It is therefore safe for diabetics. In fact, some studies are showing it actually helps reverse diabetes and metabolic syndrome by making the cells more receptive to insulin.

Xylitol and Erythritol are also naturally occurring sweeteners which are 40% less caloric than sugar, are absorbed more slowly by the body, and which do not cause the same blood sugar increases as regular sugar. They are commercially extracted from plants and trees. When used in chewing gums they have the ability to clean bacteria from teeth by preventing their binding and causing plaque. They have also been shown to wash bacteria from mucous membranes and improve immunity against infections (sugar actually has been shown to depress immunity).

Agave is as potent as honey with high amounts of fructose and glucose. Although it doesn't raise blood sugar significantly, it is not a good choice for diabetics because it is too high in fructose which will causes diabetic glycation affecting the eyes, the kidneys, and the nerves. Use it sparingly.

Splenda™ is made from dextrose (also called glucose), maltodextrin and the artificial sweetener sucralose. Sucralose is made from sugar treated with trityl chloride, as well as a bunch of chemicals only a chemist would recognize. Are you ready for this list? Acetic anhydride, hydrogen chlorine, thionyl chloride, and methanol in the presence of dimethylformamide, 4-methylmorpholine, toluene, methyl isobutyl ketone, acetic acid, benzyltriethlyammonium chloride, and sodium methoxide. This makes a sweetener unlike anything found in Nature! With that many chemicals, it's unlike anything found in the known universe! The Splenda™ Web site even states that "Although sucralose has a structure like sugar and a sugar-like taste, it is not natural." Yeah, no kidding!

The suffix *–ose* is used to name sugars, not additives. A more accurate chemical name for sucralose is trichlorogalactosucrose, but the FDA did not mandate the use of that name so the company's marketing plan named it "sucralose." The presence of chlorine is thought to be the most dangerous component of sucralose. Chlorine, as mentioned earlier in the discussion of water chlorination, is considered a carcinogen and has been used in poisonous gas, disinfectants, pesticides and plastics. The long-term effects of sucralose remain unclear.

Java Joe & Tetley

What about that morning cup of java or tea? Well, yes they are natural herbs as found in Nature, but the processing it takes to get that very concentrated cup of rich liquid energy is not natural.

Coffee beans and tea leaves are inherently high in antioxidants and are healthful herbs. When the tea is processed from green to black tea through oxidation and the coffee berry is similarly processed to become the commercial cup of coffee, problems arise. Through this processing, chemicals are further refined and even more highly concentrated to make your cup of espresso the equivalent of several cups of coffee... and you have how many shots of this?

One of the classes of concentrated chemicals in coffee are called xanthines. These chemicals are found in coffee, tea, chocolate, cola, and yerba mate' and identified as caffeine, theobromine, and theophylline among others. In women, xanthines can affect hormones and promote tissue growth resulting in fibro-cystic changes in the breasts, ovaries, and uterus. There also seems to be an associated risk of stillborn delivery for women drinking coffee during pregnancy.[6]

Caffeine causes the release of cortisol and adrenaline which can stimulate the nervous system to the point of dependence. This stimulation gives you the perception of having energy when it is actually artificially drug-induced. Many people who think they have a good energy level would actually be dog-tired if they didn't sip on their coffee-drug all day long. A single cup of morning coffee can stimulate the nervous system enough that it can keep a person lying in bed awake even 12 hours later! Cut out coffee if you have insomnia. If you are dealing with anxiety, get rid of all forms of caffeine all together.

Xanthines also act as a diuretic, causing you to urinate the precious water you've been striving to increase in your tissues. What happens at the end of the day with your water balance if you have drunk a pot of coffee, several espressos, or energy drinks? That's right - more is peed out than is taken in. You end up being dehydrated. Dehydration will exacerbate conditions like headaches, joint aches and stomach aches. Ulcers, gastritis, or other intestinal inflammation is worsened by coffee.

Besides xanthines, other molecules known as the cafestol and kahweol found in coffee beans have also been associated with health risks. These diterpene oils are known to raise the bad LDL cholesterol in humans.[7] Elevated LDL cholesterol is associated with increased rates of cardiovascular disease and stroke. These compounds are highest in coffee that is pressed and not filtered through paper. Be especially careful with French press or Turkish preparations.

Decaf coffee not the answer; it is NOT NATURAL. It is made by chemically processing beans in methylene chloride or ethyl acetate to remove the caffeine. Many decaf coffees contain an appreciable amount of xanthines as well. Do not drink decaffeinated coffee especially if you are pregnant

So, for these purposes, if you are a coffee drinker, then you should have no more than one cup of coffee or tea per day and it should be drunk with food to prevent the strong nerve stimulation. The coffee is best organic and drip-filtered through a non-bleached paper. Of course, the cream and sugar is forbidden. Non-dairy creamers are especially out; they are processed foods high in sugar and artificial flavorings. Better alternatives to coffee or tea are herbal teas including green tea if you need a bit of a boost. Green tea is loaded with powerful anti-aging antioxidants that protect us against chemicals in our environment and it can give a boost to help burn off excess fat. There are also many natural coffee substitutes made from plants which have a coffee-like flavor such as Teeccino™, Cafix™ and Pero™.

Recreational Pastimes

Surely you realize that if caffeine is out, it probably goes without saying that nicotine, alcohol and other substances used for recreational purposes (yes, marijuana too! Sorry!) are out, too. "Why? I thought a glass of red wine was beneficial." That is true to an extent, but the amount of beneficial antioxidants is actually quite low. A few glasses per week are acceptable and some studies show that in these amounts it can be health promoting. Consuming more than a drink per day or imbibing other recreational substances can affect the liver because it has to detoxify the chemical before it can be removed from the body.

Everyone is aware of the addictive qualities of alcohol, caffeine, nicotine and other recreational drugs. Their addictive nature means they have a powerful impact on the nervous system and the brain. We have waited until now to talk about eliminating them because it is important to have a solid health foundation first. When you add good food and water first there is less room, or need, for those substances which do not promote your health. Having a healthier body means you are more able to cope with the withdrawals which occur when you stopping taking these substances. Hopefully, there is now less space for boredom, and more space for inspiration. This means less time for substances which take your mind off your misery and deflate your desire to have more abundance in your life.

Where to Go from Here?

Of course if you can "Go Organic", definitely do it! If it is too expensive, which is understandable, buy it when and where you are able to afford it. If you can purchase only a few organic items due to their expense, at least make sure you are purchasing your meats or fish organically (as well butter for the rare times you have it). Animals are higher up on the food chain and accumulate toxins in their fat so it is very important that, at the very least, you buy organically raised meat for your family.

As discussed earlier, you want to eliminate all artificial chemically processed oils. Especially avoid those which are hydrogenated and partially hydrogenated and even those with concentrated processed polyunsaturated oils such as corn oil, soybean oil and canola oil. These are not found in Nature and have been processed with heat and chemicals not intended for human consumption.

It is obvious that we are not able to return to the life that our ancestors once had; foraging from the land, finding shelter in caves and living free from the chemical world in which now live. I doubt if many of us would be willing to live as our distant ancestors did, but we are creatures of Nature just as they were. The difference is that we are living in an unnatural world, created by ourselves through our own intelligence and ingenuity.

We are creating technology that is outthinking us; computers do many things we used to do manually and digital mania is taking us to new heights in construction, agriculture, transportation, communication and weaponry. Our daily lives are dependent on human inventions. They make our lives much more convenient and productive, yet in Nature we would not find them. Even modern medicine, designed to heal the body, doesn't represent Nature with its use of synthetic drugs, chemical treatments and surgeries although many of them have proven to be life-saving. The question to ask is: how many of us would need these medical interventions if we had been on Nature's Intended Path all along?

This doesn't mean our conveniences are bad, it means only that they are just that - conveniences. Our homes are constructed by means of advanced engineering and contain man-made chemicals. Our cars are designed to move us around faster and more efficiently. Our designer clothes and hygiene products keep us looking our best. Our chemically-enhanced foods with preservatives and microwave cooking make eating fast and simple. Our cell phone infatuation makes communication effortless.

Despite these conveniences, we humans are still not robots and creatures of technology, we are children of Nature. We are made from the very same substances that make up the earth, the plants, the trees and the animals. We are more Earth than we are technology, and for that reason, we will find the answers we are seeking by returning to Nature.

START NOW:

- Today, eliminate what Nature has not made. In particularly, get rid of foods containing MSG, aspartame, Splenda™, artificial colors and sweeteners and any food that contains a chemical listed on the table on the following pages. Be careful with all prepared foods found in boxes, cans, packages, or those served at public facilities or restaurants because it is usually most concentrated in chemicals.

- Today, go through your kitchen and bathroom cupboards and find foods that have toxic chemicals listed on the ingredient panels. See what to avoid by consulting the table. Throw them away.

- Talk to your health-minded doctor about helping you wean from and eliminate unnecessary medications. Ask yourself how many medications you could be taking which are simply making symptoms instead of providing a cure.

- Sweeten your foods with natural sweeteners and use them sparingly. Try also using non-caloric natural sweeteners like stevia, erythritol, and xylitol.

- Cut back or eliminate stimulating substances like coffee and black tea.

- Cut back or eliminate addictive substances such as alcohol, drugs, tobacco, sugar, coffee or anything else you find addictive.

Summary: This is what I'm doing up to this point, each day adds onto the next

Day 1: **Food awareness:** Keep a diary of my foods. I am accountable.

Day 2: **Water:** Sip half my body weight in ounces throughout the day.

Day 3: **Movement:** Some exercise performed every day. Note it in my diary.

Day 4: **Regular meals:** Eat about the same time each day.

Day 5: **Vegetables and Raw Living Foods:** 50% of total weight of your food.

Day 6: **Fruit:** Up to 2 servings of locally grown fruit daily (no fruit juice).

Day 7: **Carbohydrates:** One serving per meal combined with vegetables.

Day 8: **Protein:** One serving of healthy animal protein at every meal.

Day 9: **FAT:** Eliminate bad fats and add one serving of good fat per meal.

Day 10: Grocery shopping, food preparation, condiments, and serving sizes.

Day 11: Practical food combining: Mix, match, and rotate properly.

Day 12: Dinner or lunch type meals for breakfast (MENU IN THE BACK).

Day 13: Avoid Toxic Chemicals.

[1]Ewg.org, Public Health Reports (Thornton, et al. July-Aug 2002)

[2]Ibid

[3]Jason, et al. (Lazarou et al), Incidence of Adverse Drug Reactions in Hospitalized Patients, Journal of the American Medical Association (JAMA), Vol. 279. April 15, 1998, pp. 1200-05. Also Bates, David W., Drugs and Adverse Drug Reactions: How Worried Should We Be? JAMA, Vol. 279. April 15, 1998, pp. 1216-17.

[4]Dirlewanger, Mirjam. *Am J Physiol Endocrinol Metab* 279: E907-E911, 2000; Effects of fructose on hepatic glucose metabolism in humans.

[5]Cell Metabolism March 2009; 9(3):252-64

[6]Maternal consumption of coffee during pregnancy and stillbirth and infant death in first year of life: prospective study. BMJ 2003;326:420

[7]"The cholesterol-raising factor from coffee beans, cafestol, as an agonist ligand for the farnesoid and pregnane X receptors". Molecular Endocrinology 21 (7): 1603–16

CHEMICAL TO AVOID	WHERE FOUND
alcohol	beverages
artificial sweeteners: acesulfame, aspartame, saccharin	processed foods/beverages
artificial color FD &C #	processed foods/beverages
artificial flavors	processed foods/beverages
caffeine	coffee, tea, chocolate, cola
chlorine	water supply
dioxins	burning garbage, PVC, agent orange
drugs illicit	from a drug dealer near you
fluoride	water, fluoride treatments
fructose	processed foods/beverages
heavy metal: aluminum	anti-perspirants, antacids, cookware, cans/foil
heavy metal: arsenic	treated lumber, industry runoff= soil and water
heavy metal: lead	lead paint, plumbing, batteries, industry= soil and water
heavy metal: mercury	amalgam teeth, paints, batteries, vaccines, thermometers, coal burning, = polluted soil and water = polluted fish
heavy metal: nickel	water, jewelry, dental alloys
medications unnecessary prescriptions	from a licensed physician
MSG monosodium glutamate	processed foods/beverages
hydrolyzed /textured vegetable protein (MSG)	processed foods/beverages
autolyzed yeast extract (MSG)	processed foods/beverages
nicotine	tobacco products
Olestra™	processed foods/beverages
perfluorochemicals PFC: Teflon™, Scotchgard™	nonstick pans, Gore-Tex™, furniture, carpets, stain repellent
pesticides/ herbicides	plant and animal foods
polychlorinated biphenyls PCBs	industrial chemicals and pollution/burning
preservatives: sodium nitrate/nitrite, BHA, BHT, propyl gallate	processed foods/beverages
sulfur dioxide (sulfite), glutaraldehyde	processed foods/beverages
phthalates / plastics	plastic wrap/bags, bottles/pipes, plastic containers plastic toys, cosmetics, nail polish, hair products
Splenda™ / sucralose	processed foods/beverages
Trans fats: hydrogenated fats	processed foods/beverages
Volatile Organic Chemicals: VOCs	carpet, dry wall, particle board/plywood, glues, paint/varnish
petroleum, xylene, benzene,	permanent markers, cleaning chemicals, aerosols, air fresheners, fragrances
chlorofluorcarbons CFC, formaldehyde	insect repellents, dry cleaning, cosmetics/nail polish, deodorants, propane, methane, gasoline, auto tires, vinyl curtains
white sugar	processed foods/beverages
salt: sodium chloride	processed foods/beverages

MAY BE ASSOCIATED WITH

heart disease, cancer, neurological toxicity, multiple others

neurological disorders, muscle/joint pain, headaches, cancer, allergic disorders

neurological toxicity, mood and behavior changes

eurological toxicity, mood and behavior changes

nervous system stimulant, fibrocystic changes

heart disease, carcinogenic, thyroid dysfunction, hormone dysfunction

cancer, hormone dysfunction, infertility, neurological toxicity, liver damage

too many problems to list...including causing you to go broke

osteoporosis, arthritis, cancer, infertility, neurological toxicity, Alzheimer's, thyroid dysfunc

fatty liver, diabetes, heart disease

ALL HEAVY METALS: heart disease, cancer

ALL HEAVY METALS: neurological disease ex: Alzheimer's, Parkinson's,

ALL HEAVY METALS: Cerebral Palsy, multiple sclerosis, schizophrenia

ALL HEAVY METALS: Lowered IQ, developmental delays, mental retardation, autism, behavioral disorders like ADD and ADHD

multiple cross reactions

neurological disorders, muscle/joint pain, headaches, allergic disorders, asthma

neurological disorders, muscle/joint pain, headaches, allergic disorders, asthma

neurological disorders, muscle/joint pain, headaches, allergic disorders, asthma

heart disease, cancer, neurological toxicity, multiple others

abdominal cramping/ diarrhea, unknown

cancer, hormone dysfunction, infertility

cancer, hormone dysfunction, neurological disorders, autoimmune disease

cancer, hormone dysfunction, neurological disorders, autoimmune disease

hormone dysfunction and infertility

gastrointestinal symptoms, skin irritations,allergic reactions, palpitations, anxiety, mood changes

heart disease, cholesterol, diabetes,obesity, Alzheimers, cancer, liver dysfunction, infertility

ALL VOCS: respiratory disease: asthma, emphysema, lung cancer

cancer

heart disease, neurological disease (MS, ALS, Parkinsons, Alzheimers, migraines)

diabetes, heart disease, multiple

blood pressure, heart disease

Day 14
Vitamins, Minerals, & Supplements

There is so much confusion about supplements: which ones to take, what dosages to take, what forms, and why to choose one over another. The health food stores can bedazzle and overwhelm someone who has not visited one before. If you don't know what you are looking for you could easily be confused and end up spending money unnecessarily on wasted nutrition.

Little do most people realize that the vitamins found naturally in your food weren't discovered until 1905. The first vitamin discovered was vitamin B1, found by William Fletcher, who was looking for the cause of the disease beriberi. This is a severe nervous system disorder which he found to be caused by a deficiency of thiamine (vitamin B1). He found that people who ate only processed rice, which is the white rice that we commonly eat today, came down with beriberi while those people eating whole grain rice (brown rice) did not. Brown rice still has the nutritious brown hull casing which is high in vitamin B1 while white rice has had this nutritious shell polished and removed. This was man's first attempt at processing food to make it more desirable to our taste buds. It marked the beginning of food processing that would be a nutritional disaster for the health of our civilization. More proof that you cannot improve on Nature!

Later in 1912 a Polish scientist, Casimir Funk, performed

additional studies and named this special molecule that cured beriberi a "vitamine" after "vita" meaning life and "amine" from the compound he isolated as thiamine. He recognized that this special molecule "vitamine" provided life-giving properties. People who did not consume these molecules would be much more apt to develop this disease.

Today, the vitamins we buy from the store are not extracted from Nature's foods. They are manufactured in the same way as drugs. Both drugs and vitamins are made in labs from artificial man-made chemicals. There is nothing natural about them! Even though they are made from chemicals, the synthesized result looks like the same vitamin molecule as found in Nature. The difference is that it is cheaper to synthesize vitamins from chemicals than extract them naturally. "Ka-Ching!"

Although they have the same molecular structure as the vitamins found in Nature, artificial vitamins are made from chemicals that most of us wouldn't consider guzzling down in a glass. They are made from chemicals with names such as acetone, turpentine, and coal tar. Sound healthy? Coal tar is a complex hydrocarbon with numerous chemical constituents, such as benzene, toluene, zylene, phenol, cresol, napthaline, anthracine and pitch. You may have remembered reading about some of these chemicals and their potential dangers from the table listed at the end of Day 13. Do any of these chemicals sound like something which is natural and beneficial for your health?

Land Ho! New Discoveries Await

An interesting idea to contemplate is that prior to the discovery of vitamins, they didn't exist. At least they didn't exist to us within the knowledge of the human race. They didn't exist, the same way the world used to be flat. Well that is true; the earth was considered to be flat prior to 1492; no knowledge existed to the contrary. In fact, as we obviously know now, the earth was always round, it simply took us a while before we figured it out. Prior to 1905 we had no idea there were special substances in brown rice which prevented one from getting beriberi or other nutritional deficiency diseases. We were still living on a "flat earth" regarding the world of nutrition.

Consider that researchers have just recently discovered fifteen new species of animals including salamanders, frogs and insects in the rainforests of Ecuador.[1] Even more astounding is a newly discovered "lost world" of more than forty new species deep in the solitude of a remote volcanic crater on the Pacific island of Papua New Guinea.[2] The crater was crawling with strange new species, such as fanged frogs, grunting fish, tiny bear-like creatures, a wooly rat the size of a cat and many others which have been in isolation since the volcano erupted thousands of years ago. These were animals that had previously "never existed" and were completely unknown to modern science. Even with today's advancements, it is estimated there are approximately 14 million plants and animals in the world of which we know only about 1.8 million of them.

Even though we live in the 21st century and our technology is much advanced, we still have not discovered all the animals in the world! What does that say about the microscopic world or even the chemical world which is smaller still? There still remains so much to discover, learn and understand. Simply speaking, Nature has already put it together in ready-to-eat packages in the perfect proportions of the nutritious compounds you need for healthy living. We do not need to be scientists to discover the benefits of what is already provided for us.

As time passed and we became more technologically advanced we discovered more nutrients in foods. Did that mean that they just began to exist once we discovered them? Obviously, the answer is: NO! These nutrients have always been in our foods; we simply didn't know about them until relatively recently, and interestingly, we are still discovering more phytochemicals and other nutrients in our food even today.

The point is that the beneficial micro nutrients have always been there in our foods. They are present in the exact proportions and quantities that Nature designed for us to ingest them. What discoveries are still waiting to be discovered? Do you think it's in your synthetic multi-vitamins now? Of course it's not, unless you are taking a special multivitamin made from Nature's whole foods. Will taking handfuls of man-made vitamins protect us from all the nutritional deficiencies? Not unless it has in it all nutrients discovered and not yet discovered. It is fair to say that choosing a supplement made from Nature's whole foods will ensure that you are getting the complete complement of nutrition that was intended for your body

Plant foods are our greatest connection to the living Earth. They provide the widest variety of nutritional compounds most lacking in our modern diets, substances such as vitamins, minerals, enzymes, and antioxidant bioflavonoids. Choosing to consume the muscle (meat), bones, and organs of animals is also an excellent source of these nutrients as well as amino acids. These sources are higher on the food chain, meaning they have concentrated the nutrients from plants and are an incredibly rich source of nutrition. This is a source of nutrition that a man-made multivitamin cannot duplicate. I recommend a whole food multi to my patients like which has nutrients in the proportions that Nature intended.

Rocks for Jocks 101

Some other nutritional items you may have heard about are MINERALS!! If your body were to revert to dust (or ashes, if cremated), it would weigh about 4% of your current total weight, or roughly, between four and eight pounds. This is the weight of the seven macrominerals (calcium, magnesium, potassium, sodium, sulfur, phosphorus and chlorine) and the weight of all the trace minerals: boron, chromium, cobalt, copper, fluorine, iodine, iron, germanium, lithium, manganese, molybdenum, nickel, rubidium, selenium, silicon, strontium, tin, vanadium and zinc. These minerals are all needed for the highly specialized functions of thousands of chemical reactions in your body to maintain perfect health.

Minerals are a basic ingredient in dirt! When children have cravings to eat dirt, sand, ice, chalk, cardboard, or even their own nails and hair, it's likely they have a mineral deficiency. Plants absorb these minerals from the soil and they become a part of the plant's tissues. When you get your minerals by eating plants, you are consuming them in a form that is more assimilable, or usable for your body.

The minerals in plants are called organically-bound minerals and this is a form that the body is ready to utilize. You could get your minerals from eating dirt as well, if that's what you wish. Eating dirt or sucking on rocks or iron nails can also provide minerals but they are more difficult for the body to utilize. It is also a rather gritty and yucky way to get your necessary nutrition! It would be best to let the plants do the work for you and you eat them as Nature provided in the forms of whole grains and fruits and vegetables.

Fertile Farming for Feeding Folks

Unfortunately, many farmers are growing your fruits and vegetables on soil that has been depleted of minerals. When crops are planted on the same soil season after season the minerals in the soil can become depleted. The soil needs to be nourished yearly with minerals instead of just fertilizers. Fertilizers will make the plant grow large and look healthy but it will still be lacking in vital minerals. The minerals in the soil give plants a strong immunity to help fight against bug invaders, diseases, and weeds. They also give the plant a higher degree of flavor and logically, the more minerals in the soil, the more in the plant and the more get passed ultimately to us. It is important to support local farmers who practice conscious farming and raise organic crops on soil which is rich in nutrients.

While we are on the subject of healthy farming, it is important that we do not support the production of genetically modified organisms (GMOs). I like to consider these mutant foods. Literally, scientists take the genes from one species and transplant it into the genes of another species. Yes, you read correctly; they are taking DNA from bacteria or a virus and inserting it into the DNA of plants! Does that make as little sense to you as it does to me? The result is a plant which might produce its own pesticide, a plant which can withstand the herbicides the farmer sprays on the weeds all around it, or a plant that has some other super powers. The effect on humans and animals and other crops is not yet known although the developing research does not look encouraging. There is nothing natural about genetic engineering. These practices will eventually come back to bite us.

Minerals are essential for life and their functions are numerous. If deficient in any measurable amount, the health effects can be damaging. The signs and symptoms of mineral deficiencies can be many. Some researchers have suggested that the depletion of selenium in our soil could be responsible for the increasing incidence of cancers around the world. Other examples of mineral deficiencies are fatigue from iron deficiency, osteoporosis from calcium deficiency, muscle spasms and cramps and heart arrhythmias from magnesium deficiency, and thyroid disorders from iodine deficiency. Every organ has a propensity for a specific mineral or mineral combination to maintain its primary functions. If that mineral is low, the functions of that organ will also be affected.

Some minerals are denser in weight and have been referred to as heavy metals. These are now known to have negative effects on the body. They compete for the spaces in which the healthy minerals reside inside cellular enzymes. Heavy metals will push the healthy minerals out of the cell and can cause irreversible damage, especially on nerve tissue. The toxic heavy metals I test for in my patients are lead, arsenic, mercury, nickel, aluminum, cadmium, and radioactive metals among others. Unfortunately, as our environment becomes more polluted so do our planet's waters, the soil, the plants, the animals and – naturally - so do we!

The following are the major minerals required by the human diet:

Iodine is an essential element for the thyroid gland. It is also fundamental element required by the sexual organs such as the ovaries and breasts, and for brain development in the fetus. Lack of iodine can cause goiter, or enlargement of the thyroid gland. Goiters were once much more common than they are today due to the relatively recent development of iodized table salt. Iodine absorption can be inhibited by the fluoride atom competing with it for space in our cells; this is a side-effect of the overuse of fluoride in toothpastes and in our water supply.

If your hair is thin and falling or if you have dry skin, weak nails and deep fatigue, especially in the morning, you should consult your doctor for a thyroid workup. Most conventional doctors check only TSH (thyroid stimulating hormone) to measure thyroid function. Both TSH and the active thyroid hormones Free T3 and Free T4 should be checked to make sure they fall in the middle of the reference range.

The laboratory ranges that conventional medicine uses are the reference ranges for all the "supposed" healthy people. These reference ranges are often too wide and do not catch individuals that could be experiencing low grade chronic symptoms. You want to catch imbalances before they become imbalances and start treating when the numbers are just about ready to fall out of the reference range. Ideally you want your values to fall in the middle of the range and not too close to the low or high end of it. For example, if you are measuring Free T3, the reference range is between 220-420 pg/dL and an ideal value would be about 320 pg/dL. The reference range for TSH is between 0.5 and 4.5 mIU/mL although many health-oriented physicians will begin treating a hypothyroid with nutrition or other methods when the TSH is over 3.0 mIU/mL instead of waiting until it is over 4.5 mIU/mL. Treating when the lab values are at the low and high end of the reference range is a preventative measure and beats waiting for the condition to grow worse. The extra benefit is the patient often notices an improvement in how they feel if nutritional treatment begins sooner than later

Besides iodine deficiency, thinning hair and nails can also be due to a protein deficiency or malabsorption. Check with your health-oriented doctor if you have these symptoms. The best sources of organic iodine to supply the thyroid are provided by the sea, as Nature intended, in the forms of fish and seaweed.

Iron is the base mineral for the blood. If you don't have enough iron then you can develop iron-deficiency anemia. This can result in low levels of the protein hemoglobin that requires iron for its function. Hemoglobin uses iron to carry oxygen to every cell in your body. If your iron level is low, your ability to get life-giving oxygen to your cells will be low and you will feel fatigued. Iron deficiency is common in women who lose much blood during their menstrual cycle and children who do not eat enough iron-rich foods. Foods which are high in iron are those in which the vegetarian may not be too fond of: liver, red meat, and egg yolks. It also can be found in dark green leafy vegetables, peas, beans, nuts, dried fruit (raisins, prunes, apricots) and whole-grain products.

One of the most important antioxidant minerals, **selenium**, protects against oxidation or excessive rapid aging. Free radicals are not hippies from the 1960's although there is no doubt that hippies in the 60's created lots of free radicals in their bodies at one time! Toxic environmental chemicals, drugs, alcohol, cigarette smoke, physical exertion and stress, as well as everyday natural cellular reactions create free radicals which can damage cells. Selenium combines with a protein to make a powerful cell protector and detoxifier called glutathione. This makes it a vital mineral for healthy immune function as well as a key component in eliminating viral infections.

Medical physician Dr. Hans Nieper stated in his book *The Curious Man*, "In a selenium-deficient state, the Coxsackie virus may be transformed from a benign virus into a far more virulent form that can attack the heart of infected individuals and even cause death."

Selenium has been shown to protect against various types of cancer, cardiovascular disease, strokes and heart attacks. Athletes who have suddenly dropped dead in competition due to heart failure have been shown to be deficient in selenium. This mineral is found in fish, shellfish, organ meats, egg yolks, whole grains, and garlic.

Zinc is a trace mineral that is concentrated in the sexual organs. It is essential for the sexual development of teenagers and sexual health of men as they age. If you lack your zest and zeal for sex, zoom up your zinc! It is also a vital nutrient for the health of the nervous system and if your sense of taste or smell or hearing are lacking, zinc deficiency may be the culprit. The immune system uses zinc to fight viruses and heal wounds. In conjunction with **copper** and **manganese**, it is a key building block for an enzyme called super oxide dismutase (SOD). This enzyme is found in every human cell and is a powerful antioxidant protecting against toxins and free radicals. Looking at it this way, trace minerals are actually, if indirectly, antioxidants in themselves.

Zinc is also an important mineral for the eyes to prevent cataracts and macular degeneration in the elderly. Those white spots on the fingernails can be a sign of zinc or other trace mineral deficiency. Even poor dream recall has been associated with zinc deficiency. The highest source of natural zinc is found in oysters (hence the jokes about oysters serving as an aphrodisiac). In fact, zinc is needed to maintain healthy levels of testosterone, the "humpy hormone," that is necessary for a healthy libido in both men and women. Drinking more than one alcoholic drink a night inhibits zinc and can put a fizzle in place of your sizzle. Boost your potency and immunity with foods high in zinc like oysters, seafood, liver, meat, eggs, poultry, brewer's yeast, whole-grain bread and cereals, nuts and seeds such as cashews, almonds, and pumpkin seeds.

Silica is the most abundant mineral in the earth's crust and is the main component of sandy beaches and quartz crystals. Commercially, it is used to make glass and concrete. Our bodies use this strong material to produce collagen. This is the main protein of your skin, bones, tendons and ligaments. It is an essential mineral component for the body to make healthy shining hair, long strong nails, durable bones and tendons, and silky smooth youthful skin. Silica can be acquired from green vegetables, root vegetables, alfalfa and "horsetail" herbal tea

Chromium and **vanadium** are important trace minerals which assist insulin in utilizing glucose in our diet. Optimal sugar levels are essential in managing your weight whether you are overweight or underweight. These minerals can be helpful in decreasing sugar cravings as well as balancing blood sugar drops commonly occurring a couple hours after a meal. All diabetics and those with a propensity for high and low blood sugar levels should be looking to supplement their diet with chromium and vanadium which makes insulin work more effectively. Brewer's yeast, meat, whole-grains, dried peas, beans and peanuts are all good sources and provide the necessary building blocks so insulin can be used effectively by the cells.

Sodium and **potassium** are essential electrolytes needed by every cell in your body. They are needed for your nervous system to function, your muscles to move, and your heart to beat properly. It's no good if you can't think, move, or circulate blood! Some people have a greater need for one electrolyte over the other, although more commonly we are lacking in potassium because sodium levels are so high in our processed foods. These electrolytes are also important to maintain proper water balance, to prevent high or low blood pressure and to prevent water retention, which can result in edema and swelling. Along with magnesium, potassium aids in preventing kidney stones and muscle cramps.

Sodium is really not the villain that it is made out to be. It can be especially beneficial if you are someone who has lower blood pressure (under 107/67) *and* you tend to be fatigued and feel cold in the hands and feet. In these people sodium can help to support normal blood pressure and increase energy. Natural sea salt is a great source of sodium to help raise your blood pressure and circulate the blood to your extremities.

Think of blood pressure like the water pressure in your garden hose. If the water pressure is low the sprinkler can water only a limited amount of the garden (of course if it is too high, it can damage the garden). Raising the electrolyte level by using natural sea salt (a generous pinch of salt 3-5 times daily) is an excellent way to bring support to the adrenal glands and ease both fatigue and that chilled feeling. The extra electrolytes will bring warmth to your hands and feet and charge your brain with plenty of oxygen to activate that memory.

Potassium electrolyte is best acquired through your food intake and contrary to popular belief, it is not only found in bananas. It is found in high amounts in all vegetables and fruits; eat them in abundance. Some people who have high blood pressure or who have low blood potassium can shake it on their food as a condiment in the form of salt substitute or "potassium chloride."

In fact, the Chinese government ran a study that replaced their country's standard table salt with a salt blend containing 65% sodium chloride, 25% potassium chloride, and 10% magnesium sulfate. After 12 months blood pressure had dropped an average 10 points systolic and 5 points diastolic.[3,4] Now that is impressive! What if this one simple change was mandated in all the restaurants and processed and packaged food across the country? What a simple and inexpensive change that could save lives and cuts national health care costs across the board. You too can take advantage of the cardiovascular benefits by making your own salt blend at home. Just add a salt substitute like potassium chloride to your regular sea salt. It is sold at the store under the brand name "No-Salt™" or "Nu-Salt™."

It is important to mention senior citizens specifically here. The elder population often has circulatory imbalances which often result in elevated blood pressure. Typically I recommend an increase in water and a reduction in sodium salt. These people are usually prescribed a medication by their doctor to lower their blood pressure. Commonly, when a senior patient complains of fatigue, I look at his or her electrolyte levels. Some blood pressure medications can create imbalances in potassium electrolytes and some medicines lower the blood pressure too much. My senior patients tend to feel better if the blood pressure is kept between 120/75 to 130/80 as opposed to under 110/70. That little extra pressure makes sure the entire garden is watered with life-giving oxygen and energy.

Calcium and **magnesium** are Nature's tranquilizers. They keep the nervous system in peaceful balance and the heart in rhythm. Like silica, they are essential for strong bones, but those are just a few of the many minerals that bones require. They are found in dairy products, as learned earlier, but we know also that dairy is not Nature's method for getting these minerals to animals which are no longer infants nursing. So we must look to Nature. *Where does a cow get its calcium?* That's right! The grass they eat! Adult cows don't drink milk but eat that miraculous green stuff all day. Grasses have roots that go deep in the soil and pull all the minerals up into their leaves. All green foods are high in calcium and magnesium and are excellent sources of trace minerals. Green drinks made from the wheat grass or barley grass or alfalfa leaf are one of the very highest natural sources of minerals. I suggest my personal formulation, **"Veggie Greens™."** (see Sources) Bones are another plentiful source of minerals. Yes, your doggie loves them and so should you! Sardines in a can, chicken or turkey bone broth and oxtail broth are the purest forms of natural calcium you can eat.

Vitamin Varietals

That essentially covers the necessary minerals but what about the vitamins? Vitamins are also known as enzymes or co-enzymes, and they are the final essentials needed for proper growth, optimal chemical functions, and cellular communication. Vitamins are essential for many functions, such as cellular structure, in which vitamin C helps to make collagen in tissue. They may also act as antioxidants, such as vitamins A, C and E, which reduce cellular breakdown or aging. The B vitamins are key factors in thousands of known chemical reactions needed for the cell to survive. Vitamin deficiencies resulting in severe illnesses were more common at one time than they are today, and included diseases such as scurvy (vitamin C deficiency), rickets (vitamin D deficiency), beriberi (thiamine, vitamin B1 deficiency), xerophthalmia (vitamin A deficiency) and pellagra (niacin, vitamin B3 deficiency). These days, most processed foods have synthetic vitamins added to them to prevent some of these potentially deadly deficiencies.

So is a multivitamin even necessary? Even though Nature doesn't have them growing on trees, it would be fair to say yes, it probably is necessary. Poor land management has left much farmland stripped of its minerals. As a result, our food does not usually contain the minerals we need to maintain in this toxic world. Our need for minerals is even higher than that of our ancestors because of the quantity of toxins to which we are exposed, and to and the level of stress in our daily lives. Taking any old multivitamin or multi-mineral, however, is not the answer. They are usually produced from synthetic chemicals and made as cheaply as possible to maximize profit. And these inexpensive vitamins are put together with fillers and additives which will create hard tablets that are fast and cheap to produce but which are difficult to digest.

If you are generally healthy, you should take whole food nutrition supplements to boost where your food is lacking. These are Nature's gift of whole foods concentrated into supplement form, and not the synthetic, man-made supplements. Supplements made from whole foods are some of the best daily nutrients for people who are able to digest food efficiently. If you are going to have just one supplement in addition to your Nature's Diet, make sure it is a whole food nutritional supplement. Whole foods contain the full spectrum of nutrients with all the co-factors that make them synergistically more powerful in the body. You can't improve on Nature!

There are several sources of whole food vitamins. Look for ingredients that contain several of Nature's "superfoods" because they are concentrated with natural vitamins and minerals. Sea vegetables like seaweed and kelp comes from last great repository of minerals in the world, the sea. Whole food supplements should contain ingredients like barley or wheat grass juice powder, alfalfa powder, kelp powder, beet powder, carrot powder, brown rice powder, liver powder, bee pollen, blue green algae, mineral colloids and some others. I particularly suggest the whole food multinutrient combination that I have personally formulated called "**Nature's Nutrition™**." (see Sources on where you can obtain this.)

There are some situations, however, in which a whole food

supplement may not be enough and a high quality man-made synthetic vitamin-mineral supplement can be a good option in addition to a whole food supplement. This is especially true if the individual is already showing deficiency symptoms or depressed lab values that may require extra supplementation for a period of time. This may also be the case for the very young, for people who are elderly, and for those who have a chronic illness or who do not have the ability to assimilate the nutrients from whole food as well as healthier people. People who are ailing, or who have poor digestion, may not have the energy to extract the natural chemicals from the whole food supplement effectively.

If you fall into this category, choose a synthetic multivitamin which is either in the liquid, powder, or capsule form and do a little comparison. Make sure it isn't the most expensive or the least expensive and look for those which have a higher content of trace minerals. (See the list of the recommended daily intake I suggest to my patients below). Synthetic vitamins have labels with a long list of ingredients of vitamins and minerals with their milligram amounts side by side. Often, there will be no foods or herbs listed on the ingredient list.

Nature's Front Line

There are a couple more substances you may want to consider in addition to the whole food multivitamin mineral. Fish oils have gained a lot of popularity and they can be a very good addition to a healthful diet. Remember though, these are also not natural substances; they are processed to remove the oil from the protein of the fish and thus are a concentrated food. Nature provides us with the entire fish to eat, which gives the body the full spectrum of nutrition from both protein and fats. Also, when the oil is separated from the flesh, and comes in contact with oxygen for any length of time it has a better chance of becoming rancid and creating that unpleasant, fishy odor.

Most people, no matter how hard I urge, will just not get enough of the healthy omega-3 oils by eating fish alone. Our food today is just so imbalanced by the high amount of unhealthy omega-6 oils in our diet. Because of this, I do suggest taking 2-4 grams of **fish oil** daily in addition to whatever fish you eat in your diet. Fish oils have been shown to be very beneficial for health and balance for the heart, brain, nerves, skin and hormones, as well as for children still growing and even those still developing within the womb.

Cod liver oil is a still a favorite because it has all the benefits of fish oil along with the extra benefits of vitamins A and D in their natural states; Grandmother did know best! Both vitamins A and D are essential for the immune system, skin, mucous membranes, and thousands of enzymatic reactions. Vitamin D deficiency is one of the most common deficiencies in this country as sunlight is avoided by many people who worry about skin cancer. Vitamin D is not actually a vitamin but a hormone which is involved in hundreds of important chemical reactions and is a main player in maintaining a strong immune system. Having your vitamin D levels checked is important and they should be between 60-80 ng/ml (more on this on the chapter on sunshine).

Probiotics are another wonderful starter supplement for those wanting to regain optimal health. They have names like acidophilus, bifidus and lactobacillus. These are actually living bacteria - real live bugs! These are the bacteria which live naturally in our digestive systems and perform vital digestive functions. They make essential vitamins for us and acting as part of our immune system to defend us from invaders. They boost immunity and protect us from intestinal infections, cold and flu, urinary infections, and even allergies. They even protect against the bad bacteria which promote cavities in teeth. Naturally, they exist in very high numbers in a healthy body, living in our intestines and in the mucous membranes of the eyes, nose, mouth and vagina. Their numbers are so high that you actually have more of them living in your bodies than you have HUMAN CELLS!! Trillions and trillions!

Unfortunately the greatest killers of our natural bacteria are the chemicals in our food, water, environment and the use of antibiotics. Anti-biotics, which means "against-life", actually kill off our pro-biotics ("pro-life") and can seriously deplete these very important buggers. You should never take an antibiotic unless it has been prescribed for you by your physician as it can cause more harm than good by killing off healthy bacteria. If you are on an antibiotic make sure you are taking a probiotic supplement at the same time and take it for at least a week afterwards to prevent the common side-effects antibiotics are known for. Often the daily dose of a single probiotic capsule is not enough if you are on antibiotics. You may have to take several of them per day if you are trying to keep the good bacteria populated. Many women will experience yeast infections after being on a course of antibiotics if they do not take probiotics to replenish those good bacteria which have been killed.

These good bacteria are living organisms and they should naturally reproduce in a healthy body. We should be able to maintain a healthy population of these good bacteria if we live a healthy lifestyle and eat foods high in good bacteria occasionally. Some foods which are high in these bacteria are those which are fermented, such as sauerkraut, kimchi, raw yogurt and kefir, raw apple cider vinegar, and non-filtered beer. If you purchase vegetables from a local organic farm or farmer's market you will also be getting these bacteria from the soil that remains on them.

Critters of the Earth

Organic farms also utilize beneficial bacteria to keep the soil healthy and ward off pathogenic invaders. When the soil contains high amounts of minerals and healthy bacteria the farmer can avoid the use of the pesticides commonly used in modern agriculture. This is called organic farming. In fact, a crop which attracts insects and disease and weeds is an unhealthy crop. If farmers spray these crops to keep the bugs and the weeds down, even plants which look healthy are actually unhealthy plants deficient in minerals and healthy bacteria. Much of the produce you buy from the grocer is merely a fiber-rich, nutrient-poor food that was meant to be eaten by the insects. Healthy plants are high in nutrients and can defend themselves against insects and disease. Eating healthy plants means their healthful goodness gets passed onto you.

Healthy soil is full of good bacteria which act as soldiers to keep the bad bacteria at low levels. We can gain the health benefits of these bacteria and contribute to our own immunity by eating these plants loaded with these soil-based organisms. This is why it is so important to purchase food from local growers. You can be sure the plants are richer in minerals and higher in soil-based organisms. These good bacteria will be preserved if they are not sanitized away by sterilization or cooking. It is best to lightly rinse the organic vegetables and eat them raw if possible, especially carrots and root vegetables which are grown underground where the probiotics are the most numerous.

If you have a poor diet and are being exposed to toxic chemicals in the environment, your numbers of good bacteria can dwindle. They can also be depleted if you are fighting chronic fungal, candidal, bacterial or viral infections. Even high amounts of physical and psychological stress can affect the body's chemistry and cause these good bacteria populations to decrease.

I commonly suggest my patients take a probiotic supplement a few times a week to boost those good bacterial populations which may need some reserve support. Remember, these are live little buggies and they will propagate on their own once they are established. If you are purchasing a supplement which has live bacteria in it, you should not need to take them every day for life but rather just a few days a week. In order to increase the chances that the bacteria are alive, choose to buy probiotics that are not the cheapest available and which are preferably stored in the refrigerated section.

Phyto Protection at the Rescue

One more supplement I would recommend based on Nature's healing path would be a combination of the protective antioxidants found in our plants. Plants make protective chemicals called bioflavonoids which act as antioxidant protection against the sun. These are often colorful molecules in bright reds, oranges, yellows, greens, blues and purples that give plants their lovely hues. Science is proving, after thousands of years, that there is indeed something miraculous about these little protective colorful molecules.

These antioxidants protect the plant from the intense rays of the sun. When we eat these plants, these antioxidants protect against the effects of everyday living and slow the chemical effects of aging in us as well. They protect against the free radical damage caused by the sun, from exposure to chemicals, toxins and drugs, from the tissue breakdown that occurs during exercise, and from the damage caused by our daily stress.

No doubt you have heard of one or more of these active

antioxidants. They have such names as green tea, resveratrol, milk thistle, hawthorn, curcumin, rose hips, acerola cherry, bilberry, ginkgo, pine extract, grape seed and all berry extracts which are high in oligoproanthocyanidins (OPCs). I formulated an antioxidant combination that I am of course partial and proud. The supplement is named **Phyto-Ox™** and incorporates all these antioxidants in one comprehensive serving. By getting a wide variety you are protecting yourself from many levels of oxidation.(See Sources on how to obtain Phyto-Ox™)

The list goes on and on. Yes, there are many wonderful products out there. There are also many products out there which have the support of a great deal of money and a strong marketing campaign. If you gave me a million bucks, I could create an advertising campaign to sell you on the great medicinal qualities of the dandelions in your backyard! Successful marketing can convince you you've found the best medical cure-all of all time. Yes, dandelions are great, but you should be cautious; a strong marketing campaign doesn't guarantee the quality or effectiveness of a product. It might turn out to do nothing for you, and truthfully, the pharmaceutical market is flooded with so many products that it is wise to do your homework before buying. Often the most widely hyped products will have ingredients found in a competitor's products for a lower price. Read the labels and compare quality and quantity.

The long list of supplements available can be overwhelming for any person. Keep it simple. Stick to the basics as outlined in the previous chapters: good nutrition, pure water, vigorous exercise, lightened stress, and at least a whole food supplement to fill in the empty nutritional spaces. Add in probiotics, healthy oils, and a complete antioxidant and you have a very good start for your nutritional complement. Build a solid foundation first and then add in whichever bells and whistles if you like and you will have one of Nature's finest arsenals!

Remember not to depend solely on supplements for your nutrition. This is about following Nature's plan so remember to emphasize food over supplements. They are called supplements because they "supplement" your already highly nutritious diet; not the other way around.

Take a "supplement holiday" every weekend as well. Allow your body two days per week of rest with no supplementation. This will keep your body from being overwhelmed with chemical vitamins and it will be more likely to utilize them fully when you return to them again after your weekend "holiday."

START TODAY:

- Today, invest in a whole food supplement in capsule or powdered form. I suggest my formulation Nature's Nutrition ™ (see Sources). Get rid of your cheap chemical synthetic vitamin tablets.

- If you need extra concentrated nutrients, choose a synthetic multi that is mid-range cost and comes in either a liquid, powder, or in capsulated form. Compare the label to the table on the opposite page to make sure it contains a wide spectrum of nutrients.

- If you are really going for it then look for a good quality cod liver oil, probiotics, and a complete plant-based antioxidant combination like Phyto-Ox™. (see Sources)

[1]http://www.ircf.org/2009/06/cuador-expedition-uncovers-et-like-salamander/ Expedition uncovers ET-like salamander, Alex Morales

[2]http://www.guardian.co.uk/environment/2009/sep/07/discovery-species-papua-new-guinea Lost world of fanged frogs and giant rats discovered in Papua New Guinea. Robert Booth. The Guardian, Monday 7 September 2009 A team of scientists from Britain, the United States and Papua New Guinea found more than 40 previously unidentified species when they climbed into the kilometre-deep crater of Mount Bosavi and explored a pristine jungle habitat teeming with life that has evolved in isolation since the volcano last erupted 200,000 years ago.

[3]Am J Hypertens. 2009 Sep;22(9):934-42. Epub 2009 Aug 6.

[4]Hypertens Res. 2009 Apr;32(4):282-8. Epub 2009 Feb 27

Summary: This is what I'm doing up to this point, each day adds onto the next

Day 1: **Food awareness:** Keep a diary of my foods. I am accountable.

Day 2: **Water:** Sip half my body weight in ounces throughout the day.

Day 3: **Movement:** Some exercise performed every day. Note it in my diary.

Day 4: **Regular meals:** Eat about the same time each day.

Day 5: **Vegetables and Raw Living Foods:** 50% of total weight of your food.

Day 6: **Fruit:** Up to 2 servings of locally grown fruit daily (no fruit juice).

Day 7: **Carbohydrates:** One serving per meal combined with vegetables.

Day 8: **Protein:** One serving of healthy animal protein at every meal.

Day 9: **FAT:** Eliminate bad fats and add one serving of good fat per meal.

Day 10: Grocery shopping, food preparation, condiments, and serving sizes.

Day 11: Practical food combining: Mix, match, and rotate properly.

Day 12: Dinner or lunch type meals for breakfast (MENU IN THE BACK).

Day 13: Avoid Toxic Chemicals.

Day 14: **Supplements:** Choose whole food supplements to boost health.

- VITAMINS, MINERALS, & SUPPLEMENTS -

Nutrients found in synthetic multi-vitamin for someone that needs concentrated nutrition	Daily amount I recommend to patients
vitamin A	5,000 iu
mixed carotenoids	25,000 iu
ascorbic acid vitamin C	1000 mg
cholecalciferol vitamin D3	2000 mg
mixed natural tocopherol vitamin E	400 iu
thiamin B1	50 mg
riboflavin B2	50 mg
niacin B3	200 mg
pantothenic acid B5	300 mg
pyridoxine B6	50 mg
folic acid	1000 mcg
methylcobalamin B12	1000 mcg
biotin	400 mcg
vitamin K1	100 mcg
calcium	1000 mg
magnesium	800 mg
iodine	225 mcg
zinc	30 mg
copper	3 mg
selenium	200 mcg
manganese	15 mg
chromium	200 mcg
molybdenum	100 mcg
boron	3 mg
vanadium	200 mcg
potassium	200 mg

Day 15
Sleep

Sleep is our great rejuvenator. It regenerates the wind beneath our sails, the spark in our battery, and keeps us feeling refreshed with energy. Have you noticed how simply going to bed when you are overwhelmed by stress can make everything seem much more manageable when you wake the next morning? Sleep is healing both physically and emotionally and is vital for human health.

Fatigue is one of the most common reasons for which we seek the assistance of a doctor. Often people will think that an illness is causing their fatigue. Anemia, thyroid imbalances, blood sugar fluctuations, hormone imbalances, chronic infections, and other metabolic disorders can all cause fatigue. But, as my professor once taught me in medical school, don't go looking for zebras when you have horses all around you. In other words, the most common reason for people to feel tired is the most obvious reason of all: THEY AREN'T GETTING ENOUGH HIGH-QUALITY, UNINTERRUPTED SLEEP!

Instead of sleeping soundly through the night we are often interrupted in our sleep. We are awakened by noises, subtle light in the room, children, animals, our partner's snoring, hot flashes, night sweats, or the need to go to the bathroom. These interruptions, whether once or multiple times during the night, can prevent us from fully entering all stages of sleep which are necessary keep our bodies in balance.

In order to maintain our health, we need to enter into stage one "light sleep" and progress to stage 3 "deep sleep" and come in and out of REM sleep throughout the night. REM sleep, which is the sleep in which we have dreams, is a rejuvenating sleep where emotional healing occurs. The deepest levels of stage 3 sleep are also physically rejuvenating and healing; it is then that the body regenerates bone and muscle tissues and the immune system recovers. This is why people who are sick spend so much time resting and sleeping. It is a time for the body to repair and balance itself. It is also why babies spend so much time resting as they are rapidly building muscles, bones and organs. If it's not getting uninterrupted sleep, how can your body enter into these sleep cycles and heal itself?

In Nature, everything has a cycle or rhythm. As the earth rotates and the day turns into night and back again, Nature responds. During the day, plants open their leaves and flowers to the sun and animals of the daytime become active while those of the night seek shelter to rest. In living organisms this biological clock is referred to as the circadian rhythm. This is a 24-hour cycle which influences all living things. For every aspect of Nature there is an appropriate cycle for it; nothing is active at all moments of the day. Days become night and winter becomes spring because of these cycles.

We humans have our own natural cycle which is based on the rising and setting of the sun. The natural human cycle is to wake with the rising of the sun and to go to sleep after dark. As light shines through the eyelids of a sleeping person it signals the brain to manufacture several neurotransmitters which stimulate arousal and the person begins to wake up. By evening, the light decreases and causes the pineal gland in the brain to make the hormone melatonin, which is responsible for inducing sound sleep. Melatonin also has powerful roles in immunity and tissue regeneration as it serves as a powerful antioxidant.

S S S

From Nature's perspective, a human should awaken with the light and fall asleep with the darkness. It is not appropriate for a human being to be up during the night and sleep during the day because of these circadian hormone cycles. Those who work a night shift are often more disposed to mood imbalances such as anxiety, depression, and memory lapses. These individuals are also more likely to have metabolic syndrome, resulting in obesity, high blood pressure, high lipids and high blood sugar, conditions which eventually lead to heart disease and diabetes. They are also more likely to have immune system suppression which diminishes their resistance to sickness. Those who already are challenged with an illness, especially those with immune system illnesses like cancer and autoimmune disease, should never interrupt the circadian rhythm by working nights.

Women's hormonal and menstrual cycles are influenced by the phases of the moon. (Of course men are influenced by the phases of the moon as well... you must know one or two who become werewolves once a month?) Menstruation will often be in sync with the phases of the moon as it goes from new to full. The full moon affects certain conditions: more babies are born on full moon days, and more lunatic behavior – violence and even homicide – occurs at this time of the month. (Interesting that the word "lunatic" comes from the Latin word for moon!) Because these light/darkness cycles coincide with hormonal activity, it makes sense that a woman's hormones (and a man's, too) can become unbalanced if sleep is interrupted for a period of time.

Three factors can affect all hormone balance. I refer to them as the 3 S's: SLEEP, SUGAR and STRESS. Sugar we have discussed, Stress is of utmost importance to reduce (the effect of stress on your body and how to reduce it will be saved for my next book), but SLEEP is one of the most important of all. Your sleep is influenced by neurotransmitters secreted by the brain in response to the day and night cycle. These neurotransmitters are brain hormones and can also affect other hormonal cycles such as the menstrual cycle. Regular restful sleep by itself can do wonders for periods which are out of balance, painful, heavy and accompanied by tension and moodiness. Even menopausal symptoms such as hot flashes, headaches, memory lapses, and fatigue can be relieved by balancing sleep cycles.

The first step in balancing your sex hormones, then, is to create more rhythm in your life with your sleep cycle. You can reset your circadian rhythm by going to bed the same time each night and waking the same time each morning. You also need to get enough sleep. The average adult needs between 7-9 hours a night of solid sleep. If you get less than this, it is not enough; even if you feel fine with only 4-6 hours. This is a recuperative time in which the body repairs itself and a full seven hours minimum is required.

Tossing and Turning

It is important that you have done everything necessary for your body to fall asleep and stay asleep. We wake up at night for several reasons. One reason can be low blood sugar levels. To avoid this, it is important to have eaten an evening meal about four hours before bedtime. If you wake up in the middle of the night, try eating an easily digested snack before bed. A complex carbohydrate paired with a fat is a good, easy-to-digest food that provides long lasting energy throughout the night. A piece of whole grain sprouted toast with a little nut butter or avocado spread or maybe even a little cooked potato with olive oil and avocado would do the trick. Some other good options are cooked yam or squash with coconut oil, apple sauce with kefir, or even a small bowl of soup. Any of these will ensure that the blood sugar remains balanced for the eight hours you are asleep.

Another night-time distraction, especially for men, is getting up to urinate. You can minimize this by ceasing your fluid intake a couple hours before going to bed. People on diuretic medications are advised to take them in the morning so they won't need to urinate during the night. Remember that coffee and alcohol also act as diuretics and can also interrupt your restful sleep to drain your bladder.

Because our body temperature drops during sleep, it is also important that you do not become too cold. This can also interrupt your sleep. Be sure that the temperature will be maintained at a comfortable level throughout the night. This can be an issue for couples who sleep in the same bed while one is cold and the other too warm. Some people like to sleep with the window open, which can be quite refreshing as long as their body temperatures do not fall too low. On the opposite spectrum, menopausal hot flashes can create a very uncomfortable temperature state and should be discussed with your holistic physician to learn how to treat them so you can get a good night's sleep.

It is also very important that there are no external noises to arouse your brain during sleep. I commonly will suggest to patients who are lighter sleepers to wear soft ear plugs to keep the brain quiet at night. It takes a while to get used to them, but they can be a real life saver. Sleeping while music is playing can be okay for some people; the television, on the other hand, is not a good idea. Subconscious messages entering the mind all night doesn't even sound like a good idea.

Beams and Waves

It can't be emphasized enough that a dark room is very important. The slightest amount of light penetrating through your closed eyelids causes the brain to produce neurotransmitters that can arouse you from sleep. If you have trouble sleeping at night and there is *any detectable light at all* in your sleeping space - this includes the light from alarm clocks - these brain neurotransmitters can be stimulated to wake you unnecessarily. Your room should be as dark as a cave. If it is not, eye mask blinders or a bandana can be worn over your eyes while sleeping to ensure no light stimulates the nerves to your brain.

Some people are so sensitive to electricity and EMF waves that they should not be within an arm's length of any electrical outlets or any electrical device. Keep your lamps, alarm clocks, radios and all electrical outlets and panel boxes at least an arm's length or three feet away from your body. These frequencies have also been shown to disrupt sleep. With regard to avoiding EMF waves, I have no opinion about which direction in which to align your body while sleeping. Some people advise sleeping with your head pointing North, others insist upon South, but I don't think it matters as long as you are keeping external sources of EMF waves sufficiently far from your head.

Now a word of caution here with two common beverages: coffee and alcohol. Research has shown that even small amounts of caffeine (even decaf coffee, green tea, black tea and sodas) drunk in the morning can have a stimulating effect on a sensitive person for 24 hours carrying into the next day. So, take no caffeine if you are having trouble sleeping, not even if it is 18 hours earlier. Also, if you drink alcohol as a means to sleep, you are more than likely causing more harm than good.

Alcohol prevents the body from going into REM sleep. Even

though you slept, you really didn't get the rejuvenating rest you needed. This is why people that wake the next morning after drinking can feel extremely exhausted even if they passed out like a log ten hours before! Alcohol in the evening can also drop the blood sugar while you are sleeping, causing a person to wake up unexpectedly in the middle of the night. If you are going to bed with a drink, make sure you pair it with a light snack that has some fat and complex carbohydrates to keep your blood sugar balanced.

If you are a person who works nights, all isn't lost. Of course, the ideal situation would be for you not to work while you should be sleeping, but if it is unavoidable there are a couple things that you can do. First, make sure that when you are ready to go to bed your sleeping space is as dark as a cave and as quiet as a mouse. If it's not, wear an eye mask and earplugs. During your waking hours, it would be best to fool the brain by staying in a brightly lit environment. Some people may benefit by having a light box which simulates sunshine and which provides the full spectrum of natural light even during their evening working hours. (See Sources.)

Racing and Racing

What if the mind is racing and racing? This is a good time to practice a technique which will be expanded upon in later books. This technique involves becoming completely present in the moment. Becoming present means you pull back from the thoughts that are occupying your mind and focus your complete and total attention onto yourself and the room in which you lie. The smell of the air, the warmth of the blankets, the softness of the mattress; all attention focused on your present state. Become the watcher of your breath by directing your complete attention to watching your body breathe. Watch each and every breath as it goes in and out, in and out; put every ounce of focus on your breathing. All your attention is directed to your body and your environment. When the mind starts to drift back to worries of today or tomorrow, simply say, "presence" or "focus" and bring the thoughts back to your breath and your feelings of lying in the bed. Soon, you'll find that the body naturally just drifts off to sleep. Be persistent, don't give up; this technique takes practice.

If you do not fall asleep right away, do not get up! Stay in bed, stay focused on your breath, and stay present. Continue this mental technique in a relaxed state. Although you are not really sleeping, you are actually in a very relaxed brain wave state called the alpha state. The alpha state has been shown to be almost as restorative as sleeping. Remaining in this state you will at least be getting some rest and regeneration as opposed to just being frustrated about not sleeping.

It is important that if you are tired in the morning you do not stay in bed longer to compensate for the sleep you lost. You must get yourself up at the time you intended to wake even if you are exhausted from not sleeping that night. Push through the day and DO NOT NAP! That night, go to bed at the same time you did the night before and get the body back into rhythm. Eventually the body will get into its cycle and sleep will come naturally.

Dreamland

What about dreams? This is a magical subject that could fill volumes all by itself. Wouldn't it be amazing to download a copy of the dreams we had the night before so we could sit back and watch the movie of our mind's masterpieces? Maybe some brilliant reader will invent this for us to enjoy one day. Dreams can be very valuable in providing insight to our problems and inspiring new ideas in our lives. Dreams are also how the thinking mind unravels the stresses from the day. Your dreams may make no sense to you at all because their main purpose is to heal the emotions that burdened us that day. Haven't you noticed many times that a bad day can be so nicely remedied by simply going to bed and waking up with a fresh start?

People have received great insights about themselves simply by journaling their dreams. They may not mean anything at first, but after a while, a pattern will emerge that the dreamer will begin to recognize and understand. It is highly recommended that you write about your dreams if you remember them. You may be amazed at how your daily dilemmas were being solved for you while you slept.

Waking up with the natural light is just as important as falling asleep with the rhythm of Nature. It is preferable to have natural light enter your closed eyelids in the morning to stimulate your brain neurotransmitters so you may awaken naturally. If you live away from city lights then you should have a naturally dark room at night which gives way to a naturally lit room by dawn. This is the ideal arrangement. If you wear a sleeping mask or blindfold to bed, the natural light coming through the windows in the morning should still be bright enough to pass under your mask to awaken you. If you have no windows in your room, consider an alarm that awakens you with a light bulb which gradually brightens as your waking time comes near. The Soleil Sun Alarm™ is beneficial in this situation and can be especially helpful in the darker winter months when waking up is more difficult. (See Sources)

START TODAY:

- Tonight, go to bed at the same time you plan on retiring each night. Make sure that your sleep lasts between 7-9 hours of uninterrupted quiet time.

- Make sure your tummy is satisfied and your bladder is empty. No coffee or alcohol allowed if you are having trouble sleeping.

- Snuggle your bug in a rug which is warm and cozy. Make sure your eyes are covered and your ears are muffled. Do not be within an arm's length of any electrical items like clocks, radios or lamps.

- Do not go to bed upset or worried. If your mind starts to run circles while you lie there, get present by observing your breath and become at peace with your thoughts. If you don't fall asleep, don't worry; relaxed resting and mental quietness is equally beneficial. If you awaken and can't go back to sleep, don't get up; stay in that quiet state and watch your breath until the morning.

- Keep a dream diary to take notes of the messages from the brain.

Summary: This is what I'm doing up to this point, each day adds onto the next

Day 1: **Food awareness:** Keep a diary of my foods. I am accountable.

Day 2: **Water:** Sip half my body weight in ounces throughout the day.

Day 3: **Movement:** Some exercise performed every day. Note it in my diary.

Day 4: **Regular meals:** Eat about the same time each day.

Day 5: **Vegetables and Raw Living Foods:** 50% of total weight of your food.

Day 6: **Fruit:** Up to 2 servings of locally grown fruit daily (no fruit juice).

Day 7: **Carbohydrates:** One serving per meal combined with vegetables.

Day 8: **Protein:** One serving of healthy animal protein at every meal.

Day 9: **FAT:** Eliminate bad fats and add one serving of good fat per meal.

Day 10: Grocery shopping, food preparation, condiments, and serving sizes.

Day 11: Practical food combining: Mix, match, and rotate properly.

Day 12: Dinner or lunch type meals for breakfast (MENU IN THE BACK).

Day 13: Avoid Toxic Chemicals.

Day 14: **Supplements:** Choose whole food supplements to boost health.

Day 15: **SLEEP!** The same time each night and wake the same time daily.

Day 16
Fresh Air

One can never say enough about the benefits of fresh air. Animals and plants were never found in Nature with walls and roofs confining them in stagnant air and neither should we. We were meant to breathe the fresh air and feel the warmth of the sun on our skin.

The most basic requirement of life is the need for oxygen. If our breath is cut off, we can only survive for a short time – between 3-5 minutes. It is the most important of all necessities and even mild deficiencies or excesses of this element can affect body functions. The plants are the providers of this vital source of life. The algae in the oceans alone provide 70% of the oxygen that we breathe! What happens to us if these plants dwindle and die?

Unfortunately, the quantity and quality of our oxygen supply is dwindling because our plants are dying and carbon dioxide levels are increasing. Our planet is being polluted with an overwhelming amount of carbon dioxide, which is off-gassed from our vehicles, spewed in industrial pollution and massive forest fires, as well as being created by the clear-cutting of trees and the destruction of our rain forests.

Increasing carbon dioxide levels result in increased warming of the planet. This is called the greenhouse effect. Literally, we are creating a lid that is holding in all our waste and slowly suffocating us. Liken it to global constipation! My teacher taught me, *"Only human beings are capable of causing such damage to our Mother Earth. No other creature would destroy the very Mother who gives them life. Nature herself is self-maintaining, self-replicating, self-purifying, and self-healing."*

Quality O^2

It is becoming harder and harder to find good quality air. Poor quality air means poor quality water as the clouds release contaminated rain. This is a chain reaction which affects the quality of the soil, the quality of the plants grown in that soil, the health of the animals which feed on the plants and ultimately, the health of the animals that feed on the animals. All the way up the food chain straight into your body!

Interestingly, the most toxic air is actually inside your home. According to EPA research, the air inside the typical home is on average 2-5 times more polluted than the surrounding air. In extreme cases it can be 100 times more contaminated due to the large number of synthetic chemicals in our environment; chemicals in household cleaners, carpets, particle board products, paints, stains and even gas furnaces.[1] If you are living in a new home with chemicals being off-gassed from paints and carpets, you should have several air filters operating in addition to keeping the windows open. Older homes tend to trap mold, mildew, and dust mites from accumulated dust. It is particularly important to filter your indoor air if you live in the city because of the high level of pollution. I recommend to all my patients with allergies, chronic sinus infections and asthma to have a air filters running in their bedroom, living room, and work spaces 24 hours a day.

To protect your family from these indoor contaminants, choosing an air purifier with multiple levels of filtration is highly recommended. Specifically, look for air purifiers which contain not only a HEPA filter but which also utilize other forms of filtration such as ionization, carbon, ozone and UV light to neutralize all types of air contaminants. I have done considerable research for some time to find a filter that is both effective and affordable. See the Sources in the back of the book to see my recommendations.

Saturate the Cells

Once you have access to clean oxygen, you need to get that clean oxygen into your cells. Oxygen is the fuel of life; the body cannot make energy without it. Some people are deficient in oxygen because low hemoglobin levels in their red blood cells mean their cells are not healthy enough to carry it. Oxygen deficiency can also be due to a lack of physical activity which means your lungs are not being sufficiently ventilated. Circulation and deep breathing are essential for moving the blood throughout the body and delivering the life-giving oxygen to your cells.

To offset this oxygen deficiency, you should first determine whether or not you are anemic due to a lack of iron or B vitamins. This is easily determined with a simple blood test. Increasing your activity level with exercise is an excellent way to fill your cells with oxygen. You have already been exercising since Day 3 and it is one of the best ways to regularly circulate your blood so that it may deliver oxygen to the cells as your lungs breathe in and out. And don't forget what water is: yes, it is the molecule "H^2O." The "O" stands for oxygen, which means that drinking the water as recommended in Day 2 will also increase the body's supply of available oxygen

Fill it Up With Premium O^2

In addition to physical exercise, simple breathing exercises can also be done daily to supersaturate the cells and increase your blood oxygen levels. Conscious deep breathing from deep down in the belly in the evening or early morning outdoor air is not only healing, but also a relaxing and invigorating routine to include in your day's routine. When you begin practicing these exercises please be seated; excess oxygen can make you dizzy and in danger of falling over if you are standing.

In a sitting or lying position, choose a comfortable and quiet location, preferably out of doors, to do this exercise:

1) Start by exhaling until there is no air left to exhale. That means that you will be squeezing tightly and contracting your stomach muscles to get out the last little bit of air.

2) Then, take a slow, deep breath for the count of seven. Yes, seven! Pull it from way down deep and make sure you are pulling it from the diaphragm and not just your upper chest. That is a long time to inhale but keep pulling in air until can't take in any more. Expand that tummy and rib cage and then when you think you can't get in one more bit of air in your lungs try to suck in just a little more.

3) Hold it tight now, sit up straight, relax your shoulders and your chest. Relax the muscles of the body and hold it for seven whole seconds and then release.

4) Release and exhale for seven full seconds forcefully blowing out all the air until there is not another bit of air left in the lungs. When it seems that you have blown out every last bit, blow out one more time.

5) Repeat the process by inhaling deeply and slowly for a count of seven.

After a couple cycles relax, let go and sit there quietly and breathe normally. You will notice that your entire body is in a state of complete calm and peace. This is the perfect moment to become present in your environment and just observe the world around you without letting unnecessary thoughts or worries enter your mind. If you meditate, it is also a perfect little exercise to do prior to your meditation.

Sit there and enjoy this incredible feeling of deep relaxation. In fact, this is one of the best ways to calm a body which is anxious or hyper, and it can be done just about anywhere or at any time you need to create more tranquility. Go ahead and try it the next time you are in a traffic jam or get in a spat with someone... it works! When you get better at this technique you can increase the number of cycles you repeat further oxygenating the blood.

[1]epa.gov

START TODAY:

- A home air filter is highly recommended especially if you live in the city, in a new home with chemical fumes or in an old home with mildew and dust accumulation. Filters are especially valuable for people living with allergies, chronic sinus infections or asthma. (See Sources)

- Practice breathing exercises daily to hyper-oxygenate your blood. This is great for increasing energy levels and calming stress.

Summary: This is what I'm doing up to this point, each day adds onto the next

Day 1: **Food awareness:** Keep a diary of my foods. I am accountable.

Day 2: **Water:** Sip half my body weight in ounces throughout the day.

Day 3: **Movement:** Some exercise performed every day. Note it in my diary.

Day 4: **Regular meals:** Eat about the same time each day.

Day 5: **Vegetables and Raw Living Foods:** 50% of total weight of your food.

Day 6: **Fruit:** Up to 2 servings of locally grown fruit daily (no fruit juice).

Day 7: **Carbohydrates:** One serving per meal combined with vegetables.

Day 8: **Protein:** One serving of healthy animal protein at every meal.

Day 9: **FAT:** Eliminate bad fats and add one serving of good fat per meal.

Day 10: Grocery shopping, food preparation, condiments, and serving sizes.

Day 11: Practical food combining: Mix, match, and rotate properly.

Day 12: Dinner or lunch type meals for breakfast (MENU IN THE BACK).

Day 13: Avoid Toxic Chemicals.

Day 14: **Supplements:** Choose whole food supplements to boost health.

Day 15: **SLEEP!** The same time each night and wake the same time daily.

Day 16: **BREATHE!** Filter your air and breathe deeply.

Day 17
Sunshine

Since the very beginning of my studies, I was taught by my teachers that the sun is the source of ALL LIFE on this planet. The sun shines for a very important reason - without it we would all die. Absolutely nothing would survive. Nothing! Plants capture the sun's energy in their leaves- in little green packages called chlorophyll. When light strikes the chlorophyll it utilizes the sun's energy to combine water and carbon dioxide to make food for the plant through a process called photosynthesis. The plant then delivers the sun's energy to all those animals which eat it. A big plate of veggies is the equivalent of a big plate of sunshine! If there were no plants, animals would have nothing to eat. In humans, the rays of the sun are essential to transform vitamin D in our skin, and stimulate serotonin in our brain. If the sun wasn't essential for us, Mother Nature would have us living in darkness.

Sunbathing has become controversial, especially in the past few years. The biggest issue concerns excessive exposure to the sun and the predisposition of some people to skin cancers as a result. This is particular concern for those with fair skin who become sunburned easily.

Those who live in cloudier or darker climates further from the equator should realize that a lack of sunshine can be just as problematic as too much. A lack of sunshine can mean a lack of vitamin D. What we call vitamin D is actually not a vitamin at all but a hormone called calciferol. It is made naturally in our skin when we are exposed to sunlight. In the absence of sufficient amounts of vitamin D we are susceptible to a bone disease called rickets, as well as osteoporosis, lowered immunity, diminished cell reproduction, and numerous other illnesses. Vitamin D is an essential nutrient for thousands of metabolic and hormonal pathways. Many physicians now test for vitamin D regularly. It is an especially important test for patients with osteoporosis or cancer since low levels of vitamin D are associated with both conditions.

Recent studies have shown that only 23% of U.S. teens and adults have "sufficient" levels of vitamin D. This study found that those with dark skin complexions were almost always deficient with only 3% of this population having enough vitamin D.[1] Interestingly, this study signified people with "sufficient" levels of vitamin D. How many of these subjects actually had **optimal** levels of vitamin D? Could vitamin D deficiency be one more causal factor in the reason that rates of cancer, heart disease and diabetes are so high?

In my clinic, I regularly test the vitamin D levels of my patients. My wish is for their levels to be in the upper percentage of the reference range for vitamin D. Living here in the cloudy Pacific Northwest of Washington State, it is rare to see a patient with sufficient vitamin D levels. Actually, I cannot recall one patient who had optimal levels of vitamin D without daily supplements.

Your Own Natural Sunscreen

Your ability to tolerate the sun is determined by your individual skin pigment, which is a function of genetics and your environment. Darker skinned people have more of the chemical called melanin which acts as a natural UV block against the rays of the sun. Genetically, people with darker skin had ancestors who originated in areas closer to the equator where the sun was shining more intensely. A climate of strong daily sunshine increased production of melanin and enabled those with darker skin to survive the harsh conditions and reproduce. Those survivors passed to their offspring those genes for increased melanin production which protected them against the persistent and direct UV rays of the sun.

On the other hand, towards the poles of the globe, the people received less sunlight and there was less opportunity to manufacture vitamin D. Those people living in these darker climates needed skin which was fair enough to allow the light to enter easily and produce vitamin D. In these climates, additional melanin would be a disadvantage because it would block the little sunlight that was available. Those individuals with genes for light skin survived in the northern hemispheres and selectively passed on their genes.

Hence, those with dark skin have to be particularly mindful of vitamin D deficiency if they live in the far Northern or Southern hemispheres or areas where there is less sunlight. Those who have lighter skin must be more careful about living in the equatorial areas because they do not have the same natural protection that darker-skinned people do.

Two Sides of the Coin

Ultraviolet light from the sun comes in two main wavelengths: UVA and UVB of which 98% come from UVA. The less abundant UVB is the healthy wavelength that helps make vitamin D in your body when it shines on your skin. With only 20 minutes of midday sun exposure, your skin produces approximately 10,000 IU vitamin D. So, what happens when you go month after month without seeing the sun shine at all? You will most certainly end up with a Vitamin D deficiency. This is a situation that my fellow Northwesterners, Canadians, and Alaskans know all too well. With 10,000 units being produced by the midday sun, it is clear that Nature sees this as a vital nutrient. Compare this to the U.S. government's opinion on nutritional intake; it recommends only 200 IU for an adult per day!

Sunshine-providing UVB is essential for human life. But even though it is the healthy ray, it is also responsible for that painful red sunburn which occurs after too much fun in the summer sun. UVA waves do not cause sunburn. Serious sunburn can result in DNA damage, premature aging and skin cancer. Unlike UVB which acts on the surface of the skin, UVA penetrates deep into your skin and can cause even more damage from free radicals than UVB. Some researchers argue that UVA is directly responsible for the most dangerous form of skin cancer - malignant melanoma. For this reason it is the 'bad guy' and is the one most responsible for premature skin aging and skin cancer.

Go figure- the unhealthy UVA waves are also the same rays that are responsible for the bronzy glow of your sun kissed tan. Tanning beds have an even higher ratio of UVA to UVB waves than natural sunlight so you get tanned more efficiently. (The negative is that you are also more likely to get skin cancer without the nutritive and protective qualities of UVB). The healthy UVB waves are highest at midday and lowest in the evening and morning while UVA rays are constant all day long.

Vitamin D3 is made from UVB rays but UVA actually breaks down both vitamin D as well as vitamin A. This is Nature's method of making sure you do not get too much vitamin D from the sun. Window glass in your home or your car allows 90% of the 'bad' UVA to pass and blocks 90% of the 'good' UVB rays. This can deplete vitamin D levels, so it is recommended that you get adequate sunshine daily to get your healthy UVB rays. The trick is - DO NOT GET BURNED! If you are fair-skinned, you may never be able to be in the sun for long periods of time. Instead, expose yourself to a little sunshine bit by bit, day by day, until your body becomes accustomed to the stronger and more intense afternoon rays. If you can only tolerate a few minutes the first day... then that is ALL YOU CAN TOLERATE! Don't try to push the body beyond its ability. Spend a few minutes in the sun the first day and a few more the next, adding on a little each day. Little by little, your body will produce its own natural melanin sunscreen.

Screening the Sun

Our ancestors never had such a thing as SPF 10, 20, or 30 sunscreens; it wasn't natural. Instead, they found refuge from the sun by retreating to the shade. If there was no shade, they would cover their bodies with clothing or their skin with mudpacks to deflect the intense rays.

In fact, the increasing use of sunscreens is one of the leading reasons for the decrease in Vitamin D levels. People are scared to death to be in the sun, so they overprotect themselves from these vital rays. The SPF factor is an indicator of how well the sunscreen blocks UVB rays. If UVB is the healthy ray, then that sunscreen you cover yourself with inhibits the production of vitamin D in your body.

Interestingly, sunscreens in the United States are not required to show how well they protect against UVA as they are in some European countries. If UVA is potentially responsible for melanoma, it would make good sense to follow Europe's lead. Some researchers are even claiming that sunscreens make us *more susceptible* to skin cancers. A particular study revealed that sunscreen was helpful in preventing oxidative skin damage only during the first 20 minutes of exposure. After 60 minutes, however, skin slathered with sunscreen had more oxidative damage than unprotected skin.[2]

Sunscreens not only can overprotect us, but the chemicals they contain to block the sun can be toxic. Be especially aware of a chemical called octyl methoxycinnamate (OMC), which is toxic to cells even at low doses and which is an ingredient of almost all sunscreens. The skin is a magnificent organ which has not only the ability to sweat stuff out, but also ability to suck stuff up! Putting these sunscreens on your skin means you are literally putting it right into your bloodstream as it is absorbed.

Nature's Sun Protection

Choose instead sunscreens which more closely resemble Nature's sunscreens of clay and mudpacks. Zinc oxide and titanium dioxide are both safe minerals that can take the place of toxic chemical ingredients. There are several natural hygiene companies which manufacture sunscreens using one or both of these as the main sun-blocking agent. Read the labels and choose these sunscreens over the more toxic brands to protect yourself and your family.

Because sunscreen can be absorbed into your skin, it is also important to realize that vitamin D is an oil-soluble hormone which needs to be re-absorbed by your body once it has been produced on the surface of the skin. This absorption takes some time, and in fact can require up to 48 hours for the vitamin D oil is able to be fully absorbed and enter your bloodstream.[3]

So what happens if you wash within those two days in which

that vitamin D is being absorbed? Yep, it is washed down the drain as well! Do you see why deficiencies of this vitamin are so common? Therefore, if you shower or bathe, (and it is expected that you will) you will need to do so properly so you don't rinse off your nutrients. Which hygiene products to use will be covered soon, but simply wash yourself with plain water. That is right, bathe with pure natural water alone. Reserve the use of soap, shampoo and body washes for those areas where they are most necessary: scalp, armpits, groin, feet. The rest of the body does not need to be washed with soap; plain pure natural water is sufficient.

Remember too that during the time you spend in the sun you need to protect yourself internally. Plants make phytochemicals called bioflavonoids to protect themselves from the rays of the sun. These are powerful antioxidants that neutralize damage caused by the UV light. I recommend to my patients that they take a complex antioxidant like Phyto-Ox™ orally twice daily while spending time in the sunshine. I also recommend applying antioxidants directly to your skin before and after sunbathing for extra protection. You can do this easily by opening a capsule of Phyto-Ox™ antioxidant, mixing it in a little water to dissolve it or adding it to your moisturizer, and then rubbing it on the sun-exposed areas. (Be aware the natural plant pigments will temporarily color your skin) Any natural moisturizer with added anti-oxidants will also be effective. Do this before you apply sunblock and after sunbathing. It is just one more added protection from premature aging.

SAD Stuff

From October through February, the fall and winter seasons can be devastating for people who have seasonal affective disorder, or SAD. Here in the Pacific Northwest we tend to see quite a few patients who experience significant changes in their motivation, energy, sleep habits, and mood during the fall and winter. Even physical symptoms can be exacerbated by shorter and longer days. These people fare so much better with the sunshine and their mood will improve and clear during spring and summer.

These people can be particularly susceptible to vitamin D deficiency and should absolutely see a physician to have their levels checked. The use of sunlamps can also be helpful for these people to simulate a longer day. These lamps are most effective when utilized in the morning before sunrise and again after sunset to extend the perception of the sun's light. You should sit in front of them for about 30-60 minutes twice daily to get a positive effect. Increased light entering the retina of the eye can affect the production of the hormone serotonin and improve the moods of these folks whether it is induced by sunshine or sunlamps. (See Sources) Some manufacturers have designed lamps with special bulbs that allow you to shorten your exposure time. Shop around.

In extreme cases, I "prescribe" a vacation to a patient's favorite sunny place. Invariably, they feel more energetic and alive while they are there. This can be wonderfully beneficial for a week or two in the winter months. Patients seem to have no problem explaining to their employers or spouses that they need sunshine for a medical condition!

I urge every adult and child to get their vitamin D levels checked. Be sure your doctor orders the 25-hydroxy-vitamin D test and make sure your result falls in the optimal range of 60-80 ng/ml. If you fall below this, supplement yourself with over-the-counter vitamin D, not the prescription vitamin D from the pharmacy. This is because the prescription form is vitamin D2 called ergocalciferol, which is not an effective source. Over-the-counter vitamin D3 is called cholecalciferol and can be taken at a dosage of about 2000-5000 IUs daily for mild deficiencies. And for the record: for all those patients who ask month after month, the answer is "NO." Milk is neither an adequate source nor a recommended way of obtaining your vitamin D.

After supplementing 2000-5000 IUs daily for several months, recheck your labs to make sure that you are falling in the proper range.

[1]Jordan Lite, Scientific American, March 23, 2009

[2]Hanson Kerry M.; Gratton Enrico; Bardeen Christopher J. (2006). "Sunscreen enhancement of UV-induced reactive oxygen species in the skin". *Free Radical Biology and Medicine* **41** (8): 1205–1212.

[3]http://www.vitamindcouncil.org

START NOW:

- What to do about this epidemic of vitamin D deficiency? First, increase your sun exposure, but go slowly. Little by little, day by day, and above all do not get burned.

- Secondly, do not wear sunscreen unless you have to spend a long time in the sun. Choose healthy natural sunscreens made from zinc or titanium oxides. Protect yourself internally and externally with a complex antioxidant like Phyto-Ox™ (see Sources).

- Do not wash the vitamin D off your skin by bathing with soap for 48 hours after sun exposure.

- Have a sunlamp available to extend your days if you have a tendency to Seasonal Affective Disorder - SAD.

- Get your vitamin D levels checked and supplement with vitamin D3 if necessary. It is just that simple!

  D- D- DO IT!

Summary: This is what I'm doing up to this point, each day adds onto the next

Day 1: **Food awareness:** Keep a diary of my foods. I am accountable.

Day 2: **Water:** Sip half my body weight in ounces throughout the day.

Day 3: **Movement:** Some exercise performed every day. Note it in my diary.

Day 4: **Regular meals:** Eat about the same time each day.

Day 5: **Vegetables and Raw Living Foods:** 50% of total weight of your food.

Day 6: **Fruit:** Up to 2 servings of locally grown fruit daily (no fruit juice).

Day 7: **Carbohydrates:** One serving per meal combined with vegetables.

Day 8: **Protein:** One serving of healthy animal protein at every meal.

Day 9: **FAT:** Eliminate bad fats and add one serving of good fat per meal.

Day 10: Grocery shopping, food preparation, condiments, and serving sizes.

Day 11: Practical food combining: Mix, match, and rotate properly.

Day 12: Dinner or lunch type meals for breakfast (MENU IN THE BACK).

Day 13: Avoid Toxic Chemicals.

Day 14: **Supplements:** Choose whole food supplements to boost health.

Day 15: **SLEEP!** The same time each night and wake the same time daily.

Day 16: **BREATHE!** Filter your air and breathe deeply.

Day 17: **SUN!** Get some sunshine and optimize vitamin D levels.

Day 18
Healthy Hygiene

We learned in previous chapters that our world is jam-packed with chemicals which have not originated from Nature. These man-made chemicals can be toxic and potentially deadly as they accumulate in our food supply and in our tissues. We are starting to see the effects of these chemicals in both humans and animals as the rate of birth defects and many illnesses are increasing as never before. These illnesses include allergies, autoimmune diseases, neurological diseases, hormonal imbalances, cancers, and metabolic diseases which affect blood sugar control and cardiovascular health. Although we don't have direct control over the pollution being spewed into our environment by industry, we do have control over which chemicals we choose to put into our mouths and on our skin.

However, before we get to hygiene products, we have to make sure that our source of Nature's greatest cleanser – water - is as pure as possible. Because we have a skin that can not only excrete water but absorb it as well, the purity of the water in which we bathe should be the same as that which we drink. If you do not get your water from an underground well, you may be bathing in a public water supply that is recycled water loaded with a combination of toxic chemicals and even pharmaceutical drugs. The chlorine which is used to purify city water can combine with other chemicals in the water and create extremely toxic compounds. These have long, sinister names like disinfection byproducts (DBPs), trihalomethanes (THMs), haloacetic acids (HAA), trichloroethylene (TCE) and chloroform which are known carcinogens and may cause cancer, respiratory illnesses, liver and kidney disease and a host of other health problems.[1,2,3]

These chemicals become even more hazardous if you take a hot shower instead of a bath because the chlorine compounds vaporize and become gases. By breathing these poisons through your lungs they directly enter your blood stream.[4] These chlorine compounds can oxidize the lung tissue and worsen cases of asthma. These chemicals can also promote inflammation in your arteries as the chlorine oxidizes your blood vessels and makes them more susceptible to atherosclerosis.[5] Taking a typical shower can expose you to nearly ten times more chlorine than you would receive by drinking unfiltered tap water all day long.[6] Be especially careful of swimming in covered swimming areas that trap the chlorine gases inside for all to breathe.

The effects are numerous and the solution is simple: get a filter for your shower! If you have city water or water which has been treated with chlorine or fluoride, get an inexpensive shower filter to remove the chemicals. You will be impressed how much healthier your skin feels when it is bathed in pure water. Remember that chlorine is very drying to the skin so if you have chronically dry skin you may actually be experiencing the effect of using chlorinated water. Clean up your most important cleansing agent - your water! Please see Sources in the back of the book for recommended water filters for shower and sink.

Non-Conventional Cleaning

Conventional hygiene products like shampoo, soap, toothpaste, deodorant, lotions, hair products, cosmetics, etc. are loaded with toxic chemicals which have been shown to cause everything from infertility to neurological disorders, cancer and heart disease. Most of the problems are related to the preservatives needed to give the products a longer shelf-life. Avoid products which have chemical names listed in the table at the end of this chapter.

Start by replacing your conventional hygiene products and cosmetics for those made with natural ingredients. You can find these at a health food store or in the natural foods section of the supermarket. Look for toothpaste, soap, shampoo, and personal products of all types which contain natural or organic ingredients; these are more gentle to the body and especially more gentle for your children and pets.

Avoid products with long names you can't pronounce and in particular do not use toothpaste with fluoride, soaps and shampoos with "fragrance", antiperspirants with aluminum, or cosmetics and fingernail polishes containing phthalates. These have all been implicated in multiple health problems in humans. Remember that what you put on your skin can be absorbed into your bloodstream. Using products with artificial chemicals increases your total toxic exposure level and the implications are not fully understood yet. Don't take chances.

As stated earlier, it is important not to wash the natural protective oils from your skin with soap. Reserve the use of soap, shampoo, and body washes for those areas where it is most necessary: scalp, armpits, groin and feet. The rest of the body does not need to be washed with soap; water is sufficient. This is a healthy practice not only for ensuring the vitamin D is absorbed but also for immune protection on multiple levels.

The skin builds up a natural "acid mantle" that consists of your natural oils and creates a naturally acidic pH. This functions as a barrier to protect us from the little buggy bacterial and fungal invaders. If this is protective layer is washed off with an alkaline soap on a daily basis, it means that your body has one fewer defense mechanism against the bugs of the outside world. My mentor taught me that multiple nutrients can be lost through the skin and that if we washed with soap and water on a daily basis we could lose vitamin C and other water-soluble vitamins. Remember, that the skin is bidirectional; if the stuff can go in then stuff can also go out! He taught that soap should never be used all over the body during the winter because it would make one more susceptible to illness; current research indicates he was right.

Wash clothes in detergents which are marketed for their hypo-allergenic properties; these often will say "clear" or "free" on them.

They are devoid of scents and deodorizers. Do not use fabric softeners; they are simply more toxic chemicals and can increase your total toxic chemical burden. If you are able, the very best method would be to let Nature dry them outside in the fresh breeze- they will smell INCREDIBLE!

And be careful of household cleansers used to clean the kitchen and the bathroom. Be particularly cautious with bleach, harsh disinfectants, and sanitizers. These are some of the most toxic fumes out there. Again, you will have to do some research to find healthy alternatives, but most health food stores and grocery stores carry alternative cleansers that are biodegradable and safe for you and the environment.

Oh, and one more thing...FLOSS your teeth! It is one thing that you can safely do without worrying too much about being exposed to another chemical. The side benefit is better dental health and fresher kissing breath~ sound good?

START TODAY:

- Bathe only in water which has been purified of chlorine and other contaminants. Use a filter as suggested in Sources

- Read all labels and avoid hygiene and cleansing products whose ingredients appear in the list below. Find appropriate alternative products to take their place.

[1]Risk from exposure to trihalomethanes during shower: probabilistic assessment and control. Chowdhury S, Champagne P. Sci Total Environ. 2009 Feb 15;407(5):1570-8. Epub 2009 Jan 7

[2]Exposure to chlorination by-products from hot water uses. Weisel CP, Chen WJ. Risk Anal. 1994 Feb;14(1):101-6

[3]Estimates of cancer risk from chloroform exposure during showering in Taiwan. Kuo HW, Chiang TF, Lo II, Lai JS, Chan CC, Wang JD. Sci Total Environ. 1998 Jul 11;218(1):1-7.

[4]Ibid.

[5]Chlorination, water hardness and serum cholesterol in forty-six Wisconsin communities. Zeighami EA, Watson AP, Craun GF. Int J Epidemiol. 1990 Mar;19(1):49-58.

[6]The pool chlorine hypothesis and asthma among boys. Cotter A, Ryan CA. Ir Med J. 2009 Mar;102(3):79-82.

Summary: This is what I'm doing up to this point, each day adds onto the next

Day 1: **Food awareness:** Keep a diary of my foods. I am accountable.

Day 2: **Water:** Sip half my body weight in ounces throughout the day.

Day 3: **Movement:** Some exercise performed every day. Note it in my diary.

Day 4: **Regular meals:** Eat about the same time each day.

Day 5: **Vegetables and Raw Living Foods:** 50% of total weight of your food.

Day 6: **Fruit:** Up to 2 servings of locally grown fruit daily (no fruit juice).

Day 7: **Carbohydrates:** One serving per meal combined with vegetables.

Day 8: **Protein:** One serving of healthy animal protein at every meal.

Day 9: **FAT:** Eliminate bad fats and add one serving of good fat per meal.

Day 10: Grocery shopping, food preparation, condiments, and serving sizes.

Day 11: Practical food combining: Mix, match, and rotate properly.

Day 12: Dinner or lunch type meals for breakfast (MENU IN THE BACK).

Day 13: Avoid Toxic Chemicals.

Day 14: **Supplements:** Choose whole food supplements to boost health.

Day 15: **SLEEP!** The same time each night and wake the same time daily.

Day 16: **BREATHE!** Filter your air and breathe deeply.

Day 17: **SUN!** Get some sunshine and optimize vitamin D levels.

Day 18: **Clean Naturally:** Remove chemicals hygiene & household products.

AVOID THESE CHEMICALS!

They are commonly found in your health and beauty products and are known to cause harmful side effects- READ YOUR LABELS.

2 bromo-2 nitropropapane-1,3-diol	PABA
acrylamide	p-aminophenol
aluminum chlorohydrate	paraben
aluminum zirconium	parrafin
benzoyl peroxide	PEG-"some number"
benzyl alcohol	phenol carbolic acid
BHT, BHA	phenylenediamine
butylparaben	phthalate
dioxane	polyethylene
DMDM Hydantoin	propylene glycol
formaldehyde	petrolatum
fragrance	resorcinol
lead acetate	sodium fluoride
methyl paraben	sodium laureth sulfate
methylchloroisothiazolinone	toluene
mineral oil	triclosan
oxybenzone	triethanolamine

Day 19
Cleansing, Detoxification, Hydrotherapy, & Body Work

The true path of health is dependent not only on superb nutrition but also on regular cleansing and detoxification of the blood and organs. Our bodies are exposed to numerous toxic wastes and chemicals daily. These chemicals can be in the artificial and chemically processed foods that we stuff in our guts as well as in the thousands of environmental poisons that we encounter in our daily living space.

Contaminants from external sources, such as pesticides and herbicides, industrial pollution, gasoline and other engine fuels, plastics and Styrofoam, prescription medications, antibiotics, heavy metals, volatile organic compounds (VOCs) like formaldehyde, paint and glues, and common household cleaning solvents, can all have very serious health effects on animals and humans alike.

Besides these chemicals we are exposed to, let us also remember that our own body generates waste as well which it needs to filter and eliminate. It must eliminate carbon dioxide as well as urea and nitrogen, which are the breakdown products of food and of our own dead cells. Our hormones must be broken down and eliminated so they don't increase to unhealthy levels. Fecal wastes, which contain bacterial byproducts, also must be expelled to prevent auto-intoxication. Toxic waste overload signs can include cloudy and foul-smelling urine, swollen glands, coated tongue, bad breath and skin ailments of many types.

TTB and the Camel

All wastes, from the processed foods we eat and the thousands of chemicals we encounter, to the numerous chemicals generated by our own bodies, and including the chemical by-products of emotional stress, cumulatively creates what is called the "TOTAL TOXIC BURDEN" (TTB). Think of the total toxic burden as a camel carrying this huge load. In this case, the camel is you (let's say you are a two-humped camel instead of a one-humped camel just for fun) and the load you are carrying is the accumulation of all the chemicals found in your body.

A healthy camel can carry quite a load! A healthy camel also has the ability to lighten its load effectively. The body does this by filtering chemicals from the blood through the kidneys and liver which then eliminates them in feces, bile, urine, sweat and breath. However, if the load becomes too heavy on the camel's back, then we see the camel's legs get wobbly and are less able to support it while walking. The body's ability to eliminate becomes overburdened by this huge volume of excess toxins and its effectiveness is impaired. As a result, these toxins are circulating in greater amounts in the blood stream and negative effects start to show up on enzyme pathways, glands and hormones, nerves and brain, and the immune system.

Then, just when the camel is already wobbling and wobbling and can hardly stand one more moment, one more item burden is placed on its back, and yes... for fun we'll say it is a "straw"... and – CRUNCH!- it's the straw that broke the camel's back!

The body simply can't handle one more assault, so exposure to a seemingly harmless chemical like perfume or cigarette smoke or laundry detergent or diesel fume causes the body to respond with extreme symptom responses such as headaches or nausea. An exposure to mold or dust or pollens causes someone who's never had allergic symptoms before to be inflamed with sinusitis, swollen glands, plugged ears or even asthma. Eating out in a restaurant or having a bit of wedding cake or a treat at the carnival causes the worst digestive responses ever seen and fatigues the body for a week. Fighting with a spouse, losing a job, or getting in a fender-bender causes the skin to break out in hives, herpes or acne, and is accompanied by insomnia and anxiety. The body's load was too heavy, and the addition of one more stress to the already burdened system resulted in the symptoms, often even when someone has had a long prior history of good health.

Nature's Cleansers

In Nature, wild animals promote regular detoxification by eating an abundance of whole foods rich in nutrients such as minerals and enzymes, which act on the liver and other cells to serve as chemical detoxifying agents. They also eat plants which are high in fibers and which act as Natures' "broom" to the intestinal pathway. Simply put, they do not eat foods that are in packages, containers, cans, jars, or which are from the fast-food joint. All their food is naturally prepared, and their toxic burden is therefore lower. Needless to say, they pile fewer sticks on that camel's back!

Animals do get sick though, and they follow Nature's path when they are sick; that is correct, they stop eating. Animals will naturally abstain from food to allow their digestive systems to rest and their bodies to focus on the illness. This puts less of a burden on their digestion and more focus on detoxification and immune support. Even in sickness, we humans have lost our innate knowingness to abstain from food. Our taste buds have been so stimulated we have strong cravings for addictive flavor-intensified food and drugs and our bodies can no longer listen to Nature.

Although how to perform a fast or cleanse is the subject for my companion book: *Nature's Diet Cleanse Companion*, the concept is very interesting and can be powerful healing. As the body receives no food during a fast it says, *"Hey, I still need to eat! What are you doing, buddy?"* When it realizes that no food is coming its way it will begin to seek energy from somewhere so it turns to YOU! That is right! It will begin to eat IT'S OWN SELF... YOU!

The beauty of fasting is that the body first utilizes the non-essential tissues for energy. It breaks down excess fats, cleans plaques in the arteries and digests old scar tissue. The result is weight loss, cleaner arteries, lower cholesterol, less joint pain, a stronger immunity and a cleaner body. The benefits are incredible, but fasting can be dangerous if not done under the guidance of a professional. Absolutely, do not undergo fasting without professional supervision. See Sources in back of book to find a fasting and detoxification center near you.

There are other ways to detoxify the body besides fasting that carries less chance for harmful side effects. You can do this by optimizing the body's ability to eliminate waste on its own. The body has multiple methods with which to do this. The feces remove waste from the intestines and the kidneys clean blood through urine. The liver cleanses the blood by eliminating wastes through the bile and the lymphatic system cleanses each cell and eliminates wastes in the lymph fluid. The lungs cleanse the blood through the breath and the skin cleanses itself through sweat.

What Goes In Must Come...

Before this is discussed, it is important to realize that Nature is maintaining a balance between building up and breaking down, or more technically, between digestion and elimination. What goes in MUST COME OUT!!! Therefore, for each meal which goes in the mouth, one must come out the opposite end. In some people, this is stimulated naturally through the "gastro-colic reflex", more commonly known as the "gotta-go reflex" experienced by most people after the morning meal. Indigenous peoples and observed wild animals still have this reflex intact and healthfully have a bowel movement after each meal.

This means they have three bowel movements a day or 21 a week or 84 a month. Compare that to one every other day, or every few days, or in the extreme, the record set thus far by one of my patients, only ONE bowel movement in an entire 25 DAYS! That would be just 12 POOPS A YEAR!!! Where does all the extra waste go??? Well, it will sit there, hangout and ferment, rot, reabsorb, toxify and pollute the body...make the person feel ill... what else could it do?

Think about a piece of meat kept in a 98.6 degree environment for days on end and how it smells at the end of just one day. WHAT GOES IN MUST COME OUT! Not only come out, but also come out within a proper amount of transit time, which is about 24 hours for a healthy individual. Food eaten the day before should be out the next day. I often recommend to patient not only to track how often they are having bowel movements but also to track how long it takes for a meal to make the journey through the body. The best way to do this is to have a meal with corn kernels and then wait and see how long it takes for the kernels to reappear. Again, it should be about 24 hours.

Constipation is the most common digestive complaint in America. It is also the most preventable one if adequate water, ample vegetables and physical activity are taken in proper balance. The constipated individual also cannot ignore the urge to defecate or the body will become trained not to release. Medical studies show that up to 27% of the American population admits to suffering from constipation.[1] This would be constipation as defined by the conventional medical model, which considers a stool every three days as regular and normal. In other words, 27% of America is having as few as one or two bowel movements a week!!

Constipation and other irregularities can lead to diverticulosis, or "pockets" of fecal waste in the colon wall, which can become progressively irritated and lead to diverticulitis or irritated bowel. Advanced forms of chronic constipation can also lead to hemorrhoids, fissures, prolapsed colon, diarrhea, appendicitis, diverticulitis and the degenerative states of irritable bowel syndrome, irritable bowel disease and even cancer.

29 Feet

Digestion of our food begins in the mouth and ends with the anus. We have to take care of our teeth so they chew our food down to very small particles. Food is mixed with the saliva in our mouth which actually starts the digestion of our foods before they even hit the acids in the stomach.

The food continues down the digestive tube from the mouth to the anus for about 29 feet of travel. That is as a long as a semi-truck! The intestines are lined with many folds which have thousands of little fingers. These fingers also have even smaller fingers on them, called microfingers (or microvilli), spanning more than two thousand square feet of surface area...that is as large as a tennis court! These little fingers, or "villi", grab and absorb particles of digested food as it passes. They do this if they are functioning at their optimal level.

Amongst these microvilli in healthy persons, billions of good bacteria live and act as the first line of immune defense against the unhealthy bacteria and allergens found in our foods. These healthy or good bacteria, or probiotics, "good bugs", as they are called, crowd out the "bad bugs" and strengthen the lining of the intestines. When the good bacteria are in sufficiently high numbers the bad bacteria, yeast, viruses, parasites and fungi won't over-populate and create illness. They also make many essential vitamins, such as the B vitamins, niacin, folic acid, pyridoxine, cobalamin, biotin and vitamin K, which are important for proper health.

If one's digestive track is in an inflamed state due to unhealthy food choices and environmental chemicals, mucous can be over-produced which can be the beginning of health problems. This mucous naturally is secreted to protect the intestinal lining, but in states of inflammation, it can become thick and prevent the absorption of micro-nutrients which can result in a deficiency. On the cellular level, this thickened mucous coats the microvilli fingers inhibiting proper nutrient absorption. Without this absorption, the entire body suffers as symptoms slowly emerge, sending warning signals of impending malnourishment. All inflammation is a preliminary clue for future disease if it is not treated and resolved.

Take out the Trash

We wash our hair, scrub our body and brush our teeth...why wouldn't we clean our own septic systems? We treat our cars better than we treat our own bodies, with regular oil changes and checkups. Why not change our body's oil, clean its blood, and eliminate those excess wastes? We can actually do this by utilizing Nature's medicine in the form of botanical herbs, bark, roots, berries and leaves to cleanse and detoxify. These powerful botanical treatments are very effective method in promoting natural elimination through our detoxification organs.

Before starting any cleanse or detoxification procedure, make sure your diet is absolutely spot-on perfect. Which means you must follow Nature's dietary guidelines which you have learned in full by Day 19.

The emphasis is on ample amounts of pure water and the majority of your foods being vegetables.

Detoxification protocols should begin with intestinal cleansing. It is amazing to see the level of health which can be achieved simply by promoting the elimination of waste through the bowels. Intestinal cleansing stimulates digestion, eliminates chemical wastes and excess mucous, expels parasites and balances good bacterial populations. It is as if removing some of the load from the camel's back can help the camel get down the path much more easily. It took me many years of trial and error to perfect the formulation of my three part Digestive Detox™ intestinal cleanse. I feel it is superior to most intestinal cleanses on the market. (See Sources)

A human being can be constipated from days to even weeks without causing significant harm to the body but if the functions of the kidneys or liver shut down, you won't survive very long at all. It is just as important to urinate often or "pee freely" and stimulate bile flow as it is to eliminate fecal waste. After you detoxify the digestive tract for at least three weeks on the Digestive Detox™ intestinal cleanse, continue cleansing by choosing one or both of my cleanses for liver detoxification or urinary system detoxification. Again, it has taken me years of clinical trial and error to formulate a cleansing line that is powerful and effective. In addition to using these herbal cleanses, I highly recommend that you read the book, *Nature's Diet Cleanse Companion,* to learn how to perform a safe full body cleanse through diet and fasting that can be tailored to your lifestyle.

After you finish your two weeks on either the liver or the kidney-urinary system cleanse, switch to the cleanse which wasn't done and proceed with that for a couple weeks. It will take approximately two months for you to have cleansed your digestive tract, liver and kidneys. You may also choose to cleanse specifically for heavy metals especially if you have had heavy metal exposure or work in environments where there are high chemical loads. Farmers, welders, painters, construction workers, auto workers and those who are exposed to smoke of any kind are at higher risk for heavy metals

Maximizing the function of your organs means that they will be more effective in eliminating wastes in the future. Remember, use it or lose it! Circulation is life and stagnation is death. These organs need to be running at top shape for the blood to remain free of the poisons to which we are constantly exposed. If our organs do not circulate our blood and excrete their own specific fluids, we will get stopped up just like the toilet in your bathroom! You know what happens then, one stinky rotten mess! (Not to mention an expensive plumbing bill!)

Happy Hydro

Besides fasting and utilizing the botanical cleanses, there are other forms of detoxification which are also quite effective. Anything that will make the body sweat is excellent to remove toxins stored in the glands, skin and fat tissues. The Finnish folk know this and have been using saunas for a long time to promote health.

Through sweating, the body can expel chemical toxins in the fatty layers below the skin. The sauna treatment can expel fat-soluble toxins you have carried with you most of your life, compounds such as petrochemicals, paints, solvents, plastics, cleaning agents, pesticides, xeno-estrogens and even heavy metals. Sauna treatments are my treatments of choice for individuals with multiple chemical sensitivities. These individuals are so sensitive to the world around them they react adversely to chemicals in the environment to which other people are tolerant. This type of patient can be very difficult to treat because they may even have side effects to the very treatment that is supposed to help them. Almost all drugs and even natural medicines taken internally can cause reactions. Saunas are a good way for them to begin detoxification without the side effects other therapies may cause.

I also really like the use of saunas for acute illnesses like colds and flu. The heat raises the temperature of the body and promotes circulation. The increased heat promotes chemotaxis of the white blood cells, allowing them to move through the body more easily to capture and kill invaders. If you can make a steam bath in your sauna, add essential oils like eucalyptus, peppermint, lemon, thyme and others to open up the respiratory passages and bring relief to that stuffy, nasty cold.

Any sauna or steam bath will do the trick as long as it gets you sweating. Infrared saunas are becoming popular because a person can stay in them longer without the heat becoming too uncomfortable. High heat for an extended time can really wear a weak or sickly person out. Take it easy if you are ill. Start slowly and work your way up in time as you get accustomed to the treatment. Also, make sure you replenish the body's electrolytes after sweating profusely with a pinch of sea salt in a full glass of water.

Saunas are best done in cycles where the first cycle is to raise the body temperature to the point of sweating. Once you are sweating, rinse the body in a cool shower or bath and rub it with friction massage. After doing this for a few minutes in the cool water, jump back into the sauna until you are sweating again and then back to the cool water again. Do this back and forth at least three times. When you are finished you will feel like a Finn! (Well, maybe… no guarantees there - ask a Finn what it feels like to be one before you make any comparisons!) The body will vibrate and pulsate as the revitalized blood pumps through it with excellent circulation.

Circulation is Life

The same effect on the blood's circulation can be achieved in any hydrotherapy technique that includes the alternation of hot and cold water. Time in a hot tub followed by a cool bath or shower is another great way to stimulate circulation. For the Natural experience, go from a hot spring and jump in the cool river that flows by. Fun! (It's even more fun and more natural if you do it hippie style…in the buff- Nude! ☺

I am also an advocate of colonic hydrotherapy although it's not quite a good fit with the theme of this book since it isn't entirely natural. Colonics can increase elimination of toxins and I only recommend them if the patient is simultaneously using an herbal formula to promote bowel elimination first. If you are constipated, I would not recommend a colonic first but rather get the bowels moving with the help of an intestinal stimulant like my formula Movin Groovin ™ first. Once the bowels are moving then a colonic can do wonders to stimulate a deeper level of cleansing.

Think of a colonic like an osmotic pump. When the waste is cleared from the intestines, there is more free space for waste-saturated cells to release those wastes by the process of osmosis. It also has a stimulating affect on the gallbladder and liver, releasing their toxins into the intestine for elimination. A colonic is not just a cleansing for the large intestine, it is a cleansing for the entire body.

The lymphatic system is also cleansed when muscles contract and relax, forcing the lymph to circulate. Exercise not only helps eliminate waste through the skin by sweating, it also eliminates waste through breathing; we exhaling other wastes in addition to carbon dioxide. Remember too, that when you exercise you burn fat cells; this is where the body stores a lot of its chemical toxins. Breaking down fat cells through diet and exercise is another very excellent way to relieve the body of its TTB, its total toxic burden.

Another form of lymphatic elimination that you can perform yourself at home is "dry skin brushing", which promotes circulation of fluids within the tissues. Exfoliating the skin with a dry skin brush is another way to promote natural detoxification without herbs. Brush the skin prior to bathing, stroking the brush from the tips of the fingers and toes towards the trunk and heart. Not only does it remove the outer layer of dead skin cells, it also helps to circulate the fluids of the lymphatic system, thus creating circulation and promoting detoxification as well. These are all complementary methods to assist in cellular detoxification through improved circulation.

Align Yourself

Movement and circulation of both fluids and energy are key when considering human health. This chapter would not be complete without mentioning the importance of bodywork. There are hundreds of books written about the benefits of improved circulation and range of motion through the practices of massage, chiropractic manipulation, craniosacral and visceral manipulation, reflexology, Reiki and acupuncture, just to name a few of the dozens of types of bodywork available. The purpose of mentioning them here is to revalidate the importance of promoting circulation of both blood and nerve energy by means of these methods.

Hands-on therapy is one of the oldest forms of medicine; it pre-dates drugs and surgery by eons. In fact you instinctively give yourself bodywork whenever you hurt yourself; you immediately grab the injured area and squeeze it tightly or rub it out. Your initial response to an injury is to squeeze the tissues or rub them. Not only does bodywork improve general health by improving the body's ability to circulate, it also just feels good and can improve emotional well-being too.

These days, most people have experienced the benefit of massage, chiropractic or acupuncture for physical pains or other ailments. There are some lingering misunderstandings around bodywork that have been around since the 1920's which still prevent many people today from seeing body-work specialists who could help them greatly.

Morris Fishbein, Secretary of the American Medical Association (AMA) from 1924 to 1949, led the way with the beginning of a 50-year campaign against chiropractic medicine. There was considerable negative press about chiropractic from conventional medicine and the AMA, directed against chiropractors who, they felt, were beginning to compete with traditional allopathic medicine and thus threaten their status. The AMA even established a Committee on Quackery in the 1960's, which considered its prime mission to be the containment, and ultimately, the elimination, of chiropractic medicine. Many of the negative opinions of chiropractic and massage today are holdovers from this 50-year mass movement by the AMA to stop chiropractors.

The reputation of chiropractors being "quack bone-crackers" and massage therapists for dispensing "sexual favors" couldn't be farther from the truth. Chiropractic physicians and massage therapists undergo rigorous educational and clinical training and those professions have come a very long way. If you have never seen a chiropractor, massage therapist or other body-work specialist, and you have pain in your muscles or joints, ask around for a referral from friends or a local health food store. You may be pleasantly surprised by how well you feel after such a treatment and how much improvement you notice in your condition within a few treatments. By the way- body work is not only for physical pain- massage and adjustments promote circulation which benefits the entire body and can be beneficial for multiple symptoms. Ask your friendly chiropractor or massage therapist for details.

The Results

So, what are the results? When we improve the body's natural ability to eliminate waste, we often see chronic symptoms improve or disappear. Nature's plan is what goes in has to come out. Symptoms can be expected to improve when you take out the toxin-filled waste that is sitting there being reabsorbed.

Digestive complaints like constipation and irregularity, upset stomach and pain, heartburn, or acid stomach can all be relieved. Chronic fatigue, aches and pains such as muscle pain, joint pain, backache and headache similarly can lessen and disappear. Hormonal irregularities in both men and women resulting in weight gain or loss, menstruation difficulties, chronic yeast or bladder infections or prostatitis can be relieved through better waste elimination.

Immune imbalances causing allergies, chronic infections, sinusitis and lymph node swelling can show dramatic improvement with cleansing. Mood-related imbalances such as hyperactivity, inability to focus, sadness, nervousness, and memory insufficiency are among the neurological symptoms that can also be improved. Cleansing and detoxification are also very helpful as an adjunct to the detoxification treatment of drug, alcohol, caffeine and nicotine addictions, and for cleansing the body of pharmaceutical drug residues. Does the list sound long? It is...that is just how valuable a good cleansing program can be.

Some type of cleansing should be done as often as you change your car's oil about every 3-4 months. Even cleansing once or twice yearly for a few days is better than no cleansing at all. The change of season is a great time to start. I tell patients there is never a convenient time to cleanse. Something is always going to be happening in our busy lives. I recommend pulling out the calendar and marking the days you commit to cleansing just as you commit to any other engagement. Otherwise, it is just too easy to make another excuse for not doing it week after week. For more detailed step by step information on cleansing, information on including modified fasting, see my book on cleansing; *Nature's Diet Cleanse Companion*.

---

[1]*Higgins PD, Johanson JE Epidemiology of constipation in North America: a systematic review. Am J Gastroenterol. 2004;99:750-759.*

START TODAY:

- Pull out the calendar and mark the dates of your next detoxification cleansing. I recommend my simple 21 day intestinal cleanse Digestive Detox™ followed by the liver cleanse for two weeks and the urinary system cleanse for two weeks. All together it takes about 2 months to complete and can be repeated 6 months to a year later.

- Read the book, *Nature's Diet Cleanse Companion* and learn how to cleanse with diet and fasting.

- In your cleansing include a wide assortment of methods to further encourage waste elimination: hydrotherapies such as saunas, colonics and other cleansing modalities like skin brushing, massage, and adjustments.

Summary: This is what I'm doing up to this point, each day adds onto the next

Day 1: **Food awareness:** Keep a diary of my foods. I am accountable.

Day 2: **Water:** Sip half my body weight in ounces throughout the day.

Day 3: **Movement:** Some exercise performed every day. Note it in my diary.

Day 4: **Regular meals:** Eat about the same time each day.

Day 5: **Vegetables and Raw Living Foods:** 50% of total weight of your food.

Day 6: **Fruit:** Up to 2 servings of locally grown fruit daily (no fruit juice).

Day 7: **Carbohydrates:** One serving per meal combined with vegetables.

Day 8: **Protein:** One serving of healthy animal protein at every meal.

Day 9: **FAT:** Eliminate bad fats and add one serving of good fat per meal.

Day 10: Grocery shopping, food preparation, condiments, and serving sizes.

Day 11: Practical food combining: Mix, match, and rotate properly.

Day 12: Dinner or lunch type meals for breakfast (MENU IN THE BACK).

Day 13: Avoid Toxic Chemicals.

Day 14: **Supplements:** Choose whole food supplements to boost health.

Day 15: **SLEEP!** The same time each night and wake the same time daily.

Day 16: **BREATHE!** Filter your air and breathe deeply.

Day 17: **SUN!** Get some sunshine and optimize vitamin D levels.

Day 18: **Clean Naturally:** Remove chemicals hygiene & household products.

Day 19: **Cleansing and Detox:** Intestines, liver, kidneys, and fasting.

Day 20
SEX

Yes, I have saved the best for last. Patience is indeed a virtue.

In addition to seeking advice for losing weight, gaining more energy, and improving sleep, my patients will often seek guidance in their sex lives. They are discouraged because their sex drive isn't as powerful as it used to be or because their sexual organs are not responding as they once did. Of course, as we progress chronologically along this path called life (this is the nice phrase I use for "as we age") subtle changes occur which are to be expected. Our muscles become less taut, our hair may become gray or fall out, the skin becomes less supple, and along with these more visible effects of aging, the hormones decrease and so does sexual virility and performance.

If you're a male you may notice that your sexual desire is simply not there as it once was. Your erections may not be as firm, are more difficult to maintain, and your orgasms may be less fulfilling. Maybe you are experiencing any one of numerous urinary symptoms such as frequency, urgency, or incontinence. You may have noticed increased fat on your belly and breasts or decreasing muscle tone and strength. It can be harder to lose weight as you age and you may notice that you are more flabby and less lean and mean. You may even notice that you are less motivated or assertive. These could all be signals of declining or imbalanced levels of hormones.

If you're a menstruating female you may notice that you have mood swings during your period. You may have irregular cycles or cycles which are heavy or painful. Your body could be developing cysts in your breasts or ovaries, or growths in your uterus. Your mood might be anxious, irritable, or depressed. You may feel too tired for sex, have no urging for it at all, or find it difficult to climax.

As a menopausal female you may notice decreased breast size and your muscles being more fatty than firm. You may also experience vaginal dryness, hot flashes, night sweats and painful intercourse. Perhaps you are having sleepless nights, or a diminishing ability to recall or remember simple things that once came easily. You might also develop a weak bladder, decreased libido, and even a level of depression that causes you to withdraw and feel hopeless. These could all be signals of imbalanced or declining levels of hormones in the female.

It is natural to age of course, but it is important that you are not aging prematurely and suffering unnecessarily. Those factors that we can modify could make the difference between us being the sex machine we once were (or *thought* we were anyway!) or an impending flabby flop. First and foremost, it is important if you are noticing a drop-off in sexual function and desire that you first have a full physical with blood tests drawn. Especially if you feel this is happening at too young of an age. High blood pressure, high blood sugar, high or low cholesterol, anemia, and malfunctions of the thyroid, kidneys, and liver can all affect your sexual capacity. Make sure there is nothing else going on before you continue searching for that magic secret to cure your sexual woes.

A Lust for Laboratory Values

Regarding this blood work, be sure to ask your health-minded doctor to run a full hormone panel. Testosterone is not just a hormone for men; similarly, estrogen is not just for women. Both sexes need these in proper amounts to ensure a healthy sex life and reproductive system. If you are a male you want your doctor to check your testosterone levels (checking both total testosterone and free testosterone), DHT, DHEA-sulfate, and estradiol. If you are a female, your doctor should measure estradiol (both total estradiol and free estradiol), progesterone, testosterone, and DHEA-sulfate.

Both sexes should check thyroid hormones and salivary cortisol levels. (see Sources for salivary cortisol testing) Again, I also recommend checking that other hormone called 25-hydroxy vitamin D while you're undergoing these other tests. Have the blood drawn in the morning when hormone imbalances are commonly found and have subsequent draws done at the same time of the day. If you are a female who still menstruates, have your blood drawn between the 19th and the 23rd days of your cycle and have subsequent draws at the same time of month as the original blood draw.

When your doctor evaluates your lab values they should pay particular attention to those values which are not only flagged as high or low but also to those which are considered to be "high-normal" or "low-normal." For my patients I look out for values which fall in the "middle" of the reference range. If the value is close to either the high end the low end but not actually outside the reference range it is called high-normal or low-normal, and I treat these as if they are out of range already. More likely than not, if the patient continues living as they are, without making any lifestyle changes, he or she is going to be out of range within the next couple years anyway.

For example, if someone has blood glucose of 97 mg/dL and the range is 65-99, I start treating the person for elevated blood sugar right away – the same day. I don't recommend waiting until the labs say you are diabetic to treat the problem. We want to catch the imbalance while we can still use diet and natural treatments to have a positive impact on the body. So, if your doctor won't spend the time to look at each lab value individually, take your labs home and do the work yourself. Do the research on the internet; look up the meaning of each test and what you need to do to help heal yourself if you are borderline high or low. If your physician isn't being a detective with your lab values, you may even want to find a new physician who does take the time to look for these early imbalances.

The one exception with my method of examining the median of the reference range is with hormones. For hormones levels, I like to see my patients in the upper 25% of the reference range as opposed to right in the middle. This would point to a person who has a hormone level which is robust for his or her age rather than one which is pitiful and plummeting. For example, if the range for a given hormone is between 50 and 100 pg/nL, I would like to see my patient's somewhere between 85 and 100 pg/nL. The exceptions to this would be estrogen and DHT in males where the lower levels are desired and elevated testosterone in females where moderate levels are desired. Consult the list at the end of this chapter to find the ideal ranges for male and female hormones.

Down Down Down

In Nature, we are not unlike the animals and their sexual cycles. Female animals come into "heat" at which point they are fertile and sexually receptive. Women come into ovulation approximately two weeks after the first day of menstrual bleeding. At this time they are most fertile and more likely to be sexually receptive or interested. (It is a commonly understood joke that men must be in their "ovulation cycle" all the time because they are always sexually interested. For the record, men do not ovulate; it was just a joke.)

In Nature, as animals age their hormone levels decline making them less fertile and incapable of reproducing. So it is with humans. As we move past our twenties and into the thirties, forties and beyond, our hormones decrease slowly year by year. Although this decline is perfectly natural, we don't want them to plummet before their expected time. This can happen for many reasons. As outlined in this book, nutrition is a key component to keep hormone levels strong. Even if your hormone levels are good, chemical toxins from the environment can block their beneficial effects.

These toxins are called xenoestrogens, and they are chemicals which resemble estrogen but they do not provide the benefits of estrogen to the body. These estrogen-like chemicals are not produced by Nature and are toxic to all living things. Xenoestrogens are by-products of our chemical-filled, industrialized world and are considered responsible for stimulating estrogen receptors in both men and women.

Examples of xenoestrogens are pesticides, herbicides, medication residues, plastic residues from food and drinks containers, some cosmetics, cleaning agents, household chemicals, food additives and so on. These toxins can trick your body into thinking they are hormones when actually they just fill the spaces of the good guys with none of the positive effects. They have been linked to endometriosis, PMS, fibroids, breast and ovarian cysts, acne, hair loss, prostatic enlargement, and more seriously, cancers of the male and female sexual organs.

It is important to remind you once again to consume only organic animal products. The standard grocery store sells meats and dairy products which are contain growth hormones which can negatively impact the hormones in your body. Growth hormones are given to these animals to force them to mature at an unnaturally rapid pace. When you feed these meats and dairy products to your family you could be interfering with their natural maturation process. Growth hormones in animal products have been shown to cause children to enter puberty before the age of ten!

Nature's Hormone Helpers

Nature has given us a variety of foods and herbs which can be used to address hormone imbalances. Vegetables in the cruciferous family, such as broccoli, cauliflower, Brussels sprouts, kale, cabbage, and bok choy, collards, turnips, rutabagas, radishes, mustard, horseradish, watercress and arugula are high in a chemical called indole 3 carbinol or I3C. In the body, I3C breaks down into Diindolylmethane or DIM which has been shown to balance estrogen levels and protect against the hormonal conditions mentioned above. These plants have also been much studied for their powerful anti-cancer properties. I especially recommend them in the daily diet and in supplementation form if I feel there are symptoms pointing to estrogen metabolism.

Flax seed meal, and not just the oil either, but the whole seed ground meal contains not only the beneficial oil but also a group of chemicals called lignans, plant compounds which mimic the action of the natural hormone estrogen. For this reason, they are called "phyto (plant) estrogens." If estrogen levels are too high, lignans can block them and if the levels are too low, they can supplement them. Soy contains another type of phyto-estrogen called isoflavones while red clover and alfalfa contain yet another type called coumestans. These three substances are commonly prescribed to balance estrogen in women with menopausal symptoms and menstrual complaints and in men with prostate enlargement.

Of all foods, I feel that soy receives the most debate of any of them. There has been concern that phyto-estrogens in soy could possibly affect sexual development in children and could interact negatively with testosterone levels in men. There has also been much confusion and concern about the use of soy products in women with breast cancer or ovarian cancer. So far, the research has not yet quieted these fears. If we look to Asian countries which consume high amounts of soy, we see that they actually have fewer hormone-associated symptoms and less cancer of the sex organs than in western countries. More recently, researchers have compared dozens of studies and have found that soy is primarily protective against cancer and its recurrence.[1,2,3]

I look to Nature for the answers. Phyto-estrogens are found in many types of foods besides soy such as flax seeds, sesame seeds, oats, barley, beans, lentils, yams, wheat, rice, carrots, apples, and on and on. Because Nature provides them in so many other foods which are clearly beneficial, I expect that phyto-estrogens are more likely to be protective rather than harmful. Be reasonable, however; don't become a "sappy soy-nut" and consume soy milk, soy protein powders, soy meat and soy dessert all in one day. This would far exceed what Asian cultures would eat and these foods are all highly processed. Instead, rotate phyto-estrogens as a component of your healthy Nature's Diet. For example, include 1-2 servings of edamame, tofu, tempeh, fermented soy, soy milk or flax seeds each day to support hormone balance if you have any of the hormonal symptoms mentioned previously in this chapter.

Night Caps

Hormones may also plummet, as mentioned earlier, if you are not heeding the 3S's: SLEEP, SUGAR and STRESS. First you have to be getting proper sleep. The body needs at least seven hours, if not more, of uninterrupted sleep to maintain hormone cycles. Too much sugar and carbohydrate-rich foods will throw insulin levels out of balance. Imbalanced insulin can have a negative impact on hormone levels because insulin affects fat in the body. Weight management is very important for healthy sexual activity. Finally, if you are stressing your body out you are going to activate the stress hormones, cortisol and epinephrine which will have a further depleting effect on sex hormones. More about stress in a moment.

There are other chemical reasons besides plummeting hormones which can affect sexual functioning. Both prescription and non-prescription drugs are a leading cause of decreased sexual drive and function. Many medications can negatively impact blood flow and nervous system function associated with the sexual organs. Sometimes a simple change of medication can do wonders for your sex life. The use of other chemicals like cocaine, amphetamines, pain pills such as oxycontin and vicodin, and even marijuana, alcohol, nicotine, and caffeine in low doses, can all negatively impact sexual function.

Alcohol is a ceremonial drink used around the world for connecting socially. Drinking alcohol daily however, especially if you have more than a single drink, has a negative impact on the body's chemistry. Not only does it put strain on the liver for detoxification, but it can also strongly affect hormones. Alcohol can affect the ratio of estrogen in the body resulting in estrogen dominance.

For women, this can mean irregular and painful cycles, PMS, and cystic or fibrous growths in the breast, ovaries and uterus. For men this can mean shrinking testicles, a beer belly, and "man boobs." Sounds like the superhero hunk of burnin' love every woman wants? Alcohol actually depletes testosterone so although it may give you liquid courage to approach that special someone, it also undermines your ultimate performance. Ever heard of a "whiskey willy" (or a variation of that phrase)? Alcohol, marijuana, caffeine, nicotine and other drugs affect blood flow and circulation. Blood flow is the name of the game, if you ain't flowin' you ain't growin'! Enough said?

Erectile Exercises

Another helpful tip for sexual performance is the use of Kegel exercises. Kegels are done by tightly squeezing the muscles you use to stop your urine or to hold your urine when you have to go.

Simply squeeze as tightly as you can on these muscles and HOLD for ten seconds and repeat this ten or more times a day. For men with impotence this has been as beneficial as the use of medication as it contracts and strengthens the muscles responsible for erection. Kegels can also strengthen the muscles that contract during an orgasm, making it stronger in both men and woman. Doing these exercises regularly can tone the vaginal muscles as well and they are very helpful for incontinence in both sexes.

It is thought that an excess of estrogenic chemicals in the environment is responsible for the increased number of men with enlarged prostates. Today about half of all men over the age of 50 complain of prostate symptoms like urgency, dribbling, urinating frequently, and getting up at night to urinate. Old-time doctors at one time prescribed sitz baths and prostate massages. Sitz baths are warm baths that come up to the hips to bathe the organs in warm water which helps increase circulation to that area. They are also helpful for women with menstrual cramps, as well as for men with prostate symptoms.

A prostate massage really isn't a joke invented for comedy films. At one time prostate massages were performed by doctors to relieve the prostate of fluid which had accumulated due to inflammation. I have seen patients with BPH (benign prostatic hyperplasia) respond favorably with sitz baths and prostate massage. It is equally important to be eating a nutritious Nature's Diet high in zinc. I do not advise prostate massage for those who have a confirmed diagnosis of cancer, but it can be an effective treatment for chronic prostatitis and BPH. See Sources in the back of the book for prostate massaging devices.

Don't forget the principle of "use it or lose it" either! You must remain sexually active in order to maintain the optimal functioning of your organs. This is true for both men and women. Stimulating blood flow to the genitals promotes healthy blood circulation and healthy fluid secretion. If you don't use your organs they will slowly lose their ability to function and not perform as they once did. Your organs should be healthy and you should be able to engage in sexual activity well into your advanced years.

Of course, combining all the healthy habits that Nature has outlined in this book is incredibly important because a generally healthy body means a healthy sexual body as well. Ample water, healthy servings of veggies and quality protein, exercise, supplemental nutrition from superfoods and antioxidants, and regular cleansing are all a winning formula to support a robust sexual being.

Eager Beavers

I am commonly asked, what is normal sexual function for my age? Well, as you would expect, it is not going to be the same for a twenty-year old as it is for a ninety-year old. Can you remember in eighth grade how you could get turned-on just by looking at that special someone across the room? My buddies used to joke in high school that they'd get stimulated if the wind changed direction! Well, it isn't like that forever.

It would be fair to say that sexual activity daily or multiple times daily is common for those in their twenties and early thirties. For those in their thirties and forties, activity 3-5 times a week is healthy. Consider sexual activity 2-4 times a week to be healthy in your forties and fifties. From the upper fifties and higher it depends on the couples. Some individuals have just always been more sexually active and will maintain a higher degree of activity even at an advanced age. Those that were not highly sexual to begin with will likely maintain less activity as they age. On average though, a couple having sex 1-2 times a week to every couple weeks in their sixties and seventies is healthy.

What do I mean by healthy? Well there are many benefits that sexual activity with a partner can endow. Sex is great exercise. It burns calories, promotes cardiovascular wellness, and boosts the immune system. Frequent ejaculation in young men reduces the risk of prostate cancer later in life. Sex relieves stress, improves sleep and is great pain medicine relieving the pain of headaches, joint aches, and muscle aches. During sexual activity the hormone oxytocin is released which is said to be responsible for these positive effects. It is the same hormone that is released when a mother nurses her baby; it creates the bond between mother and child. Intimacy and bonding is strengthened between the partners as well because oxytocin is released during sexual activity. This bond is powerful- be careful who you are sharing this connection with and attaching to yourself before you make the oxytocin flow!

Having sex though does not mean that every sexual event has to end with a big explosion of fireworks and the national anthem playing. The Chinese talk about the "Tao of Sex" which is the teaching of "connecting" with your partner rather than this concept of just "getting off." In this model, couples can have intercourse and experience one another without having achieved climax per se. This is especially important for males.

The loss of semen in your advanced years is thought of by Chinese medicine to be a drain upon your "Jing" and thus your longevity. Jing is the sexual essence and reproductive energy; it is rooted in the kidneys and sexual organs of every person. Production of semen in the man, and menstrual blood (or pregnancy) in the woman, are believed to place the heaviest strains on Jing. This means that it takes a great amount of your own vital energy to produce more of what was just expelled. This is energy which could otherwise be used to heal the body. Zinc, a vital trace mineral, is lost in the semen with every ejaculation. Iron, copper, calcium and other minerals are lost with the menstrual flow. If you are ejaculating often or bleeding excessively, your body will need to regenerate these levels through your diet. Excessive ejaculation and bleeding can cause mineral deficiencies which can affect the entire body.

So if you are older and you are concerned about being able to climax with your partner, do not fret. Instead of thinking that you must reach a climax, think of intercourse as a coming together of two souls. Think of it as a way to be intimate, another way of communicating, but without the grand finale fireworks you used to blow off. If you are older, take the advice of the Chinese; you may just benefit by preserving your Jing and promoting your longevity.

Head Trips and Worry Warts

It is common for psychological or emotional stressors to have an impact on libido and sexual functioning. We tend not to give our brain enough credit for how powerfully our thoughts can impact our physiology. Think about it: if a man can create an erection just by thinking about sex, doesn't it make sense that thoughts can create a physical change in the body for both the positive and the negative? This will be discussed more thoroughly in my subsequent books on the power of our minds and our thoughts on our physiology.

A common reason for which someone cannot perform sexually, especially men in this case, is that they worry too much about their performance. They worry so much about being good lovers that when the time comes, they are not able to perform at all. This is commonly seen in relationships between older men and younger women. It is also typical between partners, when one has a very high sex drive and the other does not. Performance anxiety can create tension around sex so that it becomes scary and overwhelming instead of fun and intimate.

Another common reason, one I hear especially from women, is that they just don't like the look of their nude bodies. They don't want to be seen naked, and they don't understand how anyone could be turned on by their bodies so they go out of their way to avoid sex. Interestingly, when I talk to the partners of these women, those men had no idea that this was the reason they were not having sex anymore. They thought it was something they had done or said. In their minds they didn't really give a care what physical flaws their partner had, they wanted only to be intimate again.

Every day pressures and stresses can also have an impact on a person's ability to function sexually. Financial worries, taking care of the kids and household chores, deadlines and appointments and a host of other day to day concerns can add up to create a person who is worn out at the end of the day with no room left for his or her partner. It is easy to put work and duty ahead of those people whom we love the most.

Overcoming traumas experienced in childhood can also be a difficult challenge. Terrible memories of past abuse can taint all intimate relationships in the future. Some people never associated their dislike for sex with their unhealthy and unhappy former experiences. With a supportive and patient partner, plenty of communication and even professional counseling these individuals may be able to enjoy a healthy sex life.

The saddest and most difficult to remedy is the situation I refer to as the complete disconnect. Something has happened between the couple which prevents them from having a connection not only in the bedroom but in their day to day non-sexual lives as well. These are the couples who live together but don't love together. It is a common situation with many couples today. This is a very difficult situation to overcome because usually these couples don't see the point in trying to make things better. They often don't care to put the extra energy into saving the relationship by seeking counseling to strengthen communication. Inevitably, they lead a life which is mundane and free of intimacy. The sexual connection for them is over.

Happy Healthy Hormones

It seems that every other patient I see asks me about "bio-identical" hormones these days. It is amazing how our society thinks the "magic bullet" will ease all our woes. I do use natural or bio-identical hormones in some patients, but my perspective on treating patients with natural hormones may be different than some of my colleagues. I see the body as a whole unit, not just a single organ. "You are not just a gonad with legs!" I tell my patients. Treating just your gonad and forgetting about you as a whole person is not the answer.

This means that if I only prescribe natural hormones without addressing nutritional, chemical, and stress factors I am not benefitting my patient. Simply prescribing a medication without looking at nutritional deficiencies or chemical toxin excesses or stress overload puts me in the same position as conventional Western medical practitioners. Patients come to a natural doctor because they are not happy with conventional medicine. We as holistic physicians cannot let them down by simply prescribing a hormone, sending them on their way, and thinking all will be well. We have to treat holistically.

First and foremost, we have to identify and remove the potential blocks to hormone wellness. Underlying illnesses, imbalanced lab values, chemical toxins as described above must be addressed. Second, it is important to set up a strong nutritional foundation, one robust in nutrients, which has been a major theme of this entire book. Third, a conscious effort has to be made to reduce stress. Fourth, sleep has to be balanced and regular. Then and only then will we talk about hormones.

Interestingly, if those have all been addressed, the vast majority of my patients do not need any additional hormonal intervention for their complaints and their labs prove it. It is amazing what good living can do for the human body. If my patients are still in need of hormone balancing, I will then consider prescribing a botanical combination of herbs. There are many herbal preparations on the market which address male and female hormonal imbalances. Please see your health-oriented doctor for guidance.

If after looking at both nutrition and botanical combinations and there is still not a positive response, I will prescribe bio-identical hormones. For women, I may choose estradiol, estriol, (Bi-est), testosterone, progesterone, DHEA, and pregnenolone. For men, I may choose testosterone, DHEA, pregnenolone, and maybe progesterone. Bio-identical hormones look exactly like the hormones your body makes naturally. Synthetic hormones like Premarin™, Prempro™ and Androgel™ among others, do not look like your natural hormones. Make sure you have a USP compounded natural hormone before supplementing.

Some patients will say they don't want to take hormones because they are afraid of getting cancer. I will often respond, "If natural hormones gave cancer then we would have a lot of teenagers in trouble!" It is the truth. If hormones were responsible for cancer, we would expect to see the hormone-ridden teens full of cancer. But we do not. Natural bio-identical hormones are prescribed at low doses to mimic the amount your body would secrete naturally. It is still not known whether they will have the same cardiovascular or cancer inducing side effects as the artificial hormones Premarin™ or Prempro™. At this point though, their benefit is outweighing any unproven risks.

In addition to Kegel exercises, Dr. Eugene Shippen who wrote an excellent book titled, *The Testosterone Syndrome*, recommends some men trying natural hormones to improve symptoms of impotence, especially if the hormone cream is rubbed on the scrotum or head of the penis. He says that females and males suffering from urinary incontinence and/or fecal or gas incontinence may find that low-dose testosterone cream rubbed into the area of skin between the anus and the sexual organs (perineum) can strengthen the muscles that prevent leakage. A low-dose testosterone cream with estrogen and progesterone can be administered vaginally to lessen urinary leaking and increase moistness and suppleness of the female sexual organs. Kegel exercises must be done with the hormonal application to be effective.

Hormones benefit the health of the entire body, not just its sexual functioning. As teenagers we are fully flowing with hormones and our health is robust. We have sharp brains, powerful hearts, strong bones and taut muscles. Natural hormones like testosterone, estrogen, progesterone and DHEA play a huge role in the health of all of these. Even if sexual performance doesn't need to improve, hormones can and do assist us in all these other areas.

Men and women alike may increase their wellbeing and boost their sex drive if their lab numbers indicate the need for supplementing with bio-identicals. (See table at the end of the chapter with optimal lab values.) I always test for thyroid and adrenal hormones as well. Abnormal thyroid or adrenal function can mimic the same symptoms as abnormal sex hormones. See the flowchart below to see how the hormones are interrelated and produced. Isn't it interesting that cholesterol is what all hormones are made from? Is cholesterol really the bad substance we've been taught?

For testing thyroid function I check the TSH and want it to be under 3.0 mIU/mL. I also test the "free" or active serum thyroid hormones (free T3, free T4) in my patients in addition to the TSH. I expect these values to be in the middle to upper-middle end of the reference range. Temperature readings performed on rising and again in the morning, the afternoon and the evening can also be helpful to determine glandular function. Persistent temperature above 98.8 or below 98.0 should be addressed. Lower body temperature can be associated with thyroid and/or adrenal function.

For measuring adrenal function I recommend the salivary cortisol test known as the Adrenal Stress Index. (See Sources) This is a good objective measurement of adrenal health. A simpler way to measure adrenal stress response is to measure the blood pressure and pulse. Take the blood pressure and pulse lying down, stand, and repeat the blood pressure again in thirty seconds. If the standing systolic blood pressure falls by 5 points or more from the lying value and/or the pulse increases by more than 10 points per minute then you want to talk to your doctor about supporting the adrenal glands.

That is that! What a fun topic and it will no doubt bring more fun to your life if your sexual wellness is optimized.

START TODAY:

- For today it is important that you make sure your body is at its optimal health level. Not just for maximum sexual functioning but to ensure that you are working on the side of prevention for good overall health in the future. Make an appointment with your health-minded physician's office and ask to have the following labs listed below performed. And be sure to get your blood pressure and pulses (lying and standing), temperature, and weight while you are there.

- Boost sex-healthy foods high in zinc and other nutrients. Include natural hormone balancers in your diet such as all the vegetables in the broccoli family, flax seeds, soy beans, and alfalfa (found in whole food vitamins and green drinks- see Sources.)

- Eliminate or greatly decrease alcohol and other chemicals which could be affecting the hormonal balance.

- Practice your Kegels, holding tight for 10 seconds 10 or more times daily to strengthen your sex muscles. Don't forget the old-time treatments of sitz baths and prostate massage for prostate symptoms.

- "Use it or lose it." You have to practice from your youth until your later years to keep functioning well. You do not have to reach a climax each time, the intimate connection is powerful by itself.

- Get your head in the right place. Maintain communication to determine what may be causing a disconnect between you and your partner.

- Supplement with botanical herbal enhancers and/or bio-identical hormones if your laboratory values indicate. Supplement only after the foundational nutritional and psychological areas have been addressed first.

[1]Trock BJ et al. Meta-analysis of soy intake and breast cancer risk. J Natl Cancer Inst. 2006 Apr 5;98(7):459-71.

[2]Wu AH et al. Epidemiology of soy exposures and breast cancer risk. British Journal of Cancer (2008) 98, 9– 14

[3]Guha N et al. Soy isoflavones and risk of cancer recurrence in a cohort of breast cancer survivors: the Life After Cancer Epidemiology study. Breast Cancer Res Treat. 2009 Nov;118(2):395-405. Epub 2009 Feb 17.

Females: Optimal lab levels=

Estradiol: women in their prime about 20- 400 pg/ml varying in the month due to the female cycle

Postmenopausal 3-30,

Estradiol treatment with bio-identical hormones= 50-150 pg/ml

Estradiol Free: 1.0%-2.0% of total estradiol

Progesterone: women in their prime= about 0.5-30 ng/mL= varying in the month due to the female cycle

Postmenopausal 0- 1.0, progesterone treatment with bio-identical hormones= 20-75 ng/mL

Testosterone: 40-60 ng/dL

DHEA-S: women in their prime: 150-350-mcg/dL

TSH: 0.35-2.9 mcIU/mL

Free T3: 290-370 pg/dL

Cortisol: ASI salivary test

Glucose: Fasting AM: 80-95 mg/dL; 2 hours after meal 90-105 (about 10 points higher than fasting)

Fasting AM Insulin: under 6 mcIU/mL ; 2 hours after meal 15 mcIU/mL
Vitamin D (25 hydroxy): 60-80 ng/mL

Males: Optimal lab levels=

Testosterone: men in their prime 700-1200 ng/dL,

Testosterone treatment with bio-identical hormones= 500-900 ng/dL

Testosterone free: 2.0%-3.0% of total testosterone

DHT (di-hydrotestosterone- bad testosterone): 30-50 ng/dL

Estradiol: 15-30 pg/ml

Progesterone: 0-1.2 ng/mL

DHEA-S: men in their prime: 300-450 mcg/dL

TSH: 0.35-2.9 mcIU/mL

Free T3: 290-370 pg/dL

Cortisol: ASI salivary test

Glucose: Fasting AM: 80-95 mg/dL; 2 hours after meal 90-105 (about 10 points higher than fasting)

Fasting AM Insulin: under 6 mcIU/mL ; 2 hours after meal 15 mcIU/mL
Vitamin D (25 hydroxy): 60-80 ng/mL

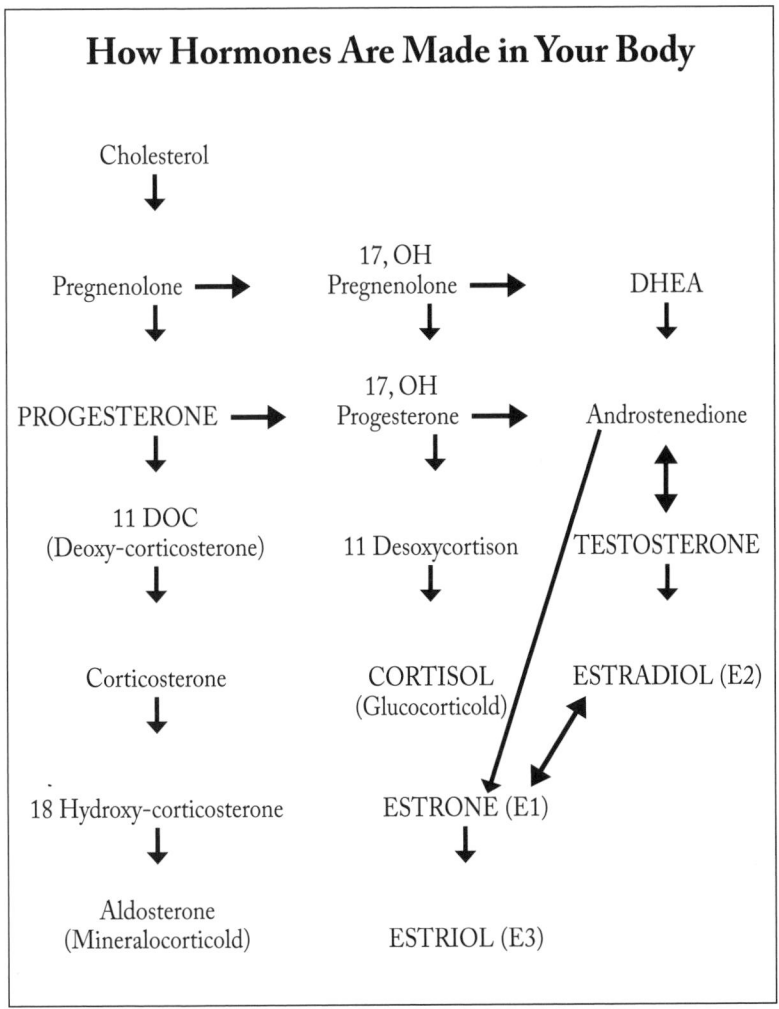

Summary: This is what I'm doing up to this point, each day adds onto the next

Day 1: **Food awareness:** Keep a diary of my foods. I am accountable.

Day 2: **Water:** Sip half my body weight in ounces throughout the day.

Day 3: **Movement:** Some exercise performed every day. Note it in my diary.

Day 4: **Regular meals:** Eat about the same time each day.

Day 5: **Vegetables and Raw Living Foods:** 50% of total weight of your food.

Day 6: **Fruit:** Up to 2 servings of locally grown fruit daily (no fruit juice).

Day 7: **Carbohydrates:** One serving per meal combined with vegetables.

Day 8: **Protein:** One serving of healthy animal protein at every meal.

Day 9: **FAT:** Eliminate bad fats and add one serving of good fat per meal.

Day 10: Grocery shopping, food preparation, condiments, and serving sizes.

Day 11: Practical food combining: Mix, match, and rotate properly.

Day 12: Dinner or lunch type meals for breakfast (MENU IN THE BACK).

Day 13: Avoid Toxic Chemicals.

Day 14: **Supplements:** Choose whole food supplements to boost health.

Day 15: SLEEP! The same time each night and wake the same time daily.

Day 16: BREATHE! Filter your air and breathe deeply.

Day 17: SUN! Get some sunshine and optimize vitamin D levels.

Day 18: **Clean Naturally:** Remove chemicals hygiene & household products.

Day 19: **Cleansing and Detox:** Intestines, liver, kidneys, and fasting.

Day 20: SEX! Balance your hormones and communicate your concerns.

Day 21
Continuing Rather Than Concluding
Treats, Wine, & Eating Out

ONGRATULATIONS! You have made it all 21 days! You have created new, positive, and healthy habits for life! I urge you not to stop now. I encourage you to make this not just a 21 day plan but a complete "change of life plan." The only way you are going to be at your optimal health is by making this "diet" a complete change of lifestyle for the rest of your life. You have done so well in improving your health; you certainly do not want to lose what you have gained by going back to your old unhealthy ways. Do your best and follow Nature's Healing Path: eat, breathe, move, think, feel, love and live in accordance with Nature.

Now that you have mastered the program for these 21 days, I challenge you to apply the daily suggestions for another 21 days. It is important to keep going. Continue and persevere so these suggestions will be locked into the brain as a long-lasting positive habit. My patients who practice this daily remark how much more energy they have and how great they feel. They look noticeably healthier and more youthful. The more you follow Nature's plan, the more it becomes your walk of life and not just some "fad diet."

A saying which has caught on and of which I am often reminded is, "We live to eat rather than eat to live." This means the most important aspect of life is to eat only food which tastes good. Your taste buds have control over your mind. They are making your food choices for you and these choices are determining the shape of your body. Now don't get me wrong… "living to eat" is very enjoyable and joy should not be sacrificed because it is very healthful emotion for the physical body. Celebrations and holidays are times at which you should certainly live to eat. For the majority of your meals however, you will be in balance if you choose to "eat to live," meaning that you choose food that is healthful for your body regardless of its taste.

If you choose to live predominantly as Nature invites you to, it should not matter if you go out to enjoy yourself once in a while. Go ahead and enjoy your meat pasta with Alfredo sauce, pepperoni pizza and beer, a delicious slice of lemon pie or a chocolate ice cream sundae once in a while. What matters instead, is how often "once in a while" becomes.

Think of it as the "90/10 compromise." In reality it would be more reasonable to call it the "80/20 compromise." But I have learned that with many patients, if I say 80/20 they will naturally cheat more and the result will be more like 70/30. So we will call it the "90/10 compromise." This means 90% of your meals are as suggested according to Nature and 10% of the meals are total wildcards. Seriously, 10% of your meals are whatever you wish to have to tickle your delight buttons! So if that means that you are eating twenty-one meals a week, (which by now you should be eating at least that many, if not more) then two of those meals you choose to eat whatever it is that you so desire. Does that make sense?

So since you did so well for 21 days, go ahead and enjoy a treat. Did you really think this was about my being the Grinch and taking away all your presents? Go ahead and enjoy! Yes, you can, no guilt, worry-free, it is one of the joys of life. Have one meal of whatever you have been really craving. Do it! Go for it! Really enjoy it and be entirely present while you eat it. Enjoy and savor every single bite; taste it fully in your mouth before you swallow.

What you might notice is that it takes less of this "comfort food" to be satisfied than it did before you started Nature's foods. Also, you may have noticed that your taste buds have changed. The old food you used to like may not taste as delicious as you had once thought it did. If chocolate chip cookies were your weakness before, you now may instead see them as tasteless dough with gritty white sugar, frothy hydrogenated oil, and embedded with fake waxy chocolate chips. Don't be surprised if your body responds strangely after not eating junk food for a while. It may even reject it with a stomach ache, vomiting or diarrhea. This is not uncommon so be prepared.

Subtle Messages

In fact, if you had been eating according to Nature since your youth, the natural bodily responses would tell you if you are eating a food which is potentially harmful to you. For example, some babies have a strong reaction to cow's milk the first time they drink it. But, since milk "does a body good" (as the ads used to say), a well-intentioned mother continues to feed her baby cow's milk. So the baby is given milk to drink even though it vomits it up over and over.

Well, our bodies are so dynamic that if you keep giving it something it doesn't want over and over, instead of continually reacting, the body finally says, *"Alright already- I give up! I can't keep reacting like this over and over. Since you're not paying any attention to me and my symptoms I might as well just stop reacting like this."* This is the point when something called TOLERANCE is reached and the symptoms stop.

A good example of tolerance can be seen with cigarette smoking. Think of the first time someone tries smoking a cigarette. The first reaction by the body is *"Cough, cough, cough, cough, cough!"* On the second try, they react with, *"cough, cough, cough."* The third time, they react with, *"cough, cough"* until finally it is just a little *"cough"* and finally.... An *"ahhhhhh..."* Tolerance is amazing stuff!

Back to the baby. Instead of reacting, the body now tolerates the milk product and the baby no longer vomits. But, tolerating it doesn't mean everything is fine. Simply because the body isn't responding with the original symptoms doesn't mean the body still wants the milk (or the cigarette). But, since you are still feeding cow's milk to the baby, the baby's body tries to send you messages in different ways. Instead of vomiting now it sends you new messages in the form of stomach aches, diarrhea, skin rashes, headaches, runny nose, or other minor symptoms. These symptoms are the body's most benign and harmless ways to try and tell you a second time, *"Stop, there is something wrong here! I'm trying to tell you to stop eating this food!"*

So as the story goes, humans don't pay attention to the body's messages very well. As the baby becomes a toddler, the parents continue to feed it milk even while the body is still screaming out, *"NO, STOP!"* After a while, the body again realizes that still nobody is listening. Instead of continuing to scream with these benign symptoms, it tries once again to adjust to the milk. It figures if you are going to keep abusing it with foods, it better find a way to calm itself. So over time these new symptoms may just go away, or you may just "grow out of it" just as the doctor said you would. The body is becoming even more tolerant. The parents are happy and the child is happy and celebrates by eating cheese and ice cream and chocolate milk.

Although the child has reached a tolerance and the symptoms are no longer present it doesn't mean the problems have disappeared. Since the underlying problem wasn't addressed, the harmless symptom may turn into a more serious condition. The runny nose, diarrhea, and rashes may now become more chronic symptoms. Now the body reacts with swollen glands, enlarged tonsils, dark circles and creases under the eyes, persistent colds or infections, chronic ear infections, throat infections and sinus infections. Now the body is screaming, *"Hey, now you better really wake up!! These problems are getting worse!"*

In response, Mom or Dad takes little Johnny to the doctor. The doctor does the exam and says, "Johnny is going to need an antibiotic for these infections." So the child is given the antibiotic and then continues to enjoy milk and cheese and yogurt. And the tonsils are swelling more and more and the ears are still getting infected every month and it seems we are never getting rid of that pesky cold. So we go back to the doctor and the doctor gives yet another course of antibiotics until the doctor finally says, "Well, those tonsils are chronically swollen and the ears are chronically infected, so let's remove the tonsils and put tubes in the ears to cure this problem." Sure enough, we get that done and the child is feeling so much better. They are not having the same chronic infections any more. They celebrate and have a pizza and ice cream sundae party.

Eventually the child grows up into a young adult who thinks he hasn't had problems with milk since childhood. He still loves pizza, chocolate milk, ice cream, and yogurt and eats it daily. Little does he know that the benign symptoms he no longer has are silently turning into a chronic disease. He wonders why he is now developing allergies to animals, pollens, dust and some foods. "Why now? I never had them before." He wonders why he is prescribed an inhaler by his doctor for the episodes of asthma he's been having. He wonders about the steroid creams prescribed to stop the itch from eczema which has become chronic. He wonders how these more serious symptoms seemingly came from nowhere. He may not even be aware that his allergy medication, the asthma medication and steroids are now additionally suppressing his immune system and putting stress on his liver.

Years go by and the middle-aged adult is diagnosed with a serious life-changing disease. Could it be that years and years of ignoring the body's messages resulted in this? Could it be the harmless symptoms deepened and become more chronic until they resulted in a serious illness? All because we didn't listen or pay attention to Nature's most benign message to us. Whether it was a simple stomachache, vomiting, diarrhea, headache, rash, nausea, fatigue, excitability, mood disturbance, stuffiness, phlegm or a runny nose; whatever the simple symptom was we ignored it. Are you suffering from symptoms which are messages sent by your body but which you ignored?

Hit the RESET Button

After twenty-one days of eating healthfully, you will have given the body proper time to reset. You may notice that many of your chronic symptoms are no longer as pronounced. Some of you may notice your symptoms have disappeared completely. You may notice that your energy is better and your sleep is deeper and your attitude is more positive. In general, the majority of my patients begin to feel positive changes in their body within two or three weeks of following Nature's Diet and lifestyle program. You may feel so good that you don't want to even "mess it up" by going back to your old ways. I have heard many patients say this and their positive health responses alone were enough to keep them from drifting off the program.

For the most of us though, we will still want to have our occasional indulgence. This is fine as long as it is kept to the 90/10 compromise.

After you have been eating so well for twenty-one days, don't be surprised if your body reacts strongly to foods which you have been avoiding. Because your body has been reset, you will be much more sensitive to your trigger foods now. When you have your meal of indulgence, the body may react with signs or symptoms within a day or two after eating. This is because the reset button has been hit and your body is now able to get through to you with the messages it has been trying to give you for years, *"Hey buddy! Stop putting that in your mouth!"*

Headaches, joint pain, muscle pain, fatigue, upset stomach, diarrhea or constipation, skin break outs, insomnia and anxiety are among a few of the messages your body might use to tell you that it didn't like what you fed it. These messages weren't being heard before because you ignored them in the beginning and the body eventually became TOLERANT. It is very important that you pay close attention to what the body is telling you this time. Be aware of these reactive symptoms you have to the food you ate. These symptoms are your body talking to you. This is your chance to make a change and not take in what the body does not want. This time, do not ignore it! Do it before it is too late and the body gives up trying to talk to you and become tolerant again.

For example, if you are enjoying pizza as your treat meal and you notice that later that evening you had stomach aches and diarrhea, it is a clear message that your body says one or more ingredients did not work well with you. Get back on your healthful eating for a week and when you are feeling better try another challenge meal with nothing but cheese (one ingredient in the pizza). If you feel fine afterwards let the body again reset for a couple days by eating healthfully as recommended. At the next challenge meal have only pizza crust. If the symptoms come back with a vengeance you will know that more than likely you were sensitive to the ingredients in the crust which is more than likely the wheat flour. By paying attention to the amount of wheat you ingest and dramatically decreasing it or by eliminating it entirely you may be surprised how much healthier you feel.

It is not always this easy to identify the offending foods. You might be someone who is reacting to their food but you can't quite identify which food is the culprit. In challenging cases like this, I recommend the IgG ELISA allergy test. This can help to identify these slow insidious allergies which could be contributing to a chronic condition. Ask your health-minded doctor to run a full panel on your blood to identify the potentially contributing foods. (see Sources)

Again, some of you may choose not to drift from the food program at all. Often, people who change their diet and lifestyle will notice they really have no cravings or desire for other foods. These people may choose to reward themselves by other means. Maybe you buy a new present for yourself, spend a day at the spa, or just some time alone. Whatever you choose, make sure you give recognition for those good things which you are doing for yourself. Giving recognition helps the brain to associate positive feelings with healthy living. Compare this to what the brain was given to associate with before. Remember how you used to feel: tired, fat, sluggish, bloated, ugly, depressed and unmotivated? Make that old picture a painful one so you never want to see it again!

Speaking of pictures, this is a good time to take a new photo of yourself. This suggestion is especially helpful for those wanting to reduce their weight. Sometimes we can't always remember how much different we looked at one time. Tape a photo of yourself at your highest weight on the fridge. Make sure it is a photo which does not bring back happy memories. It should remind of how painful that lifestyle was at times. And then put a photo of your new self or a photo of yourself when you were at your prime. This is an excellent way for your brain to make an association of the pain of one and the pleasure of the other.

Trick or Treats?

In general it is best not to buy treats and have them in the house (unless it is Halloween, of course). If you are to get something special, only do it a couple times a week and buy only as much as you will enjoy at that moment. You remember what happened to cookies that were in the cookie jar when you were little, don't you? Yeah! You ate them! Or if you weren't allowed to eat them...you snuck them. Make it difficult and labor-intensive to acquire food that is not healthy for you. Remember humans avoid pain and conserve energy and if it is more painful and requires too much energy and money to drive to the store each time you want a treat, then you won't do it.

Okay, okay, okay, I know, I know... I can hear it now...you have been aching to know, "What about chocolate?" Alright, alright, yes, you may choose to enjoy your chocolate a couple times a week as part of the 90/10 compromise if you wish. Dark chocolate would be the best for you because milk chocolate is not as healthful. If you can find chocolate made from raw cacao beans it is going to be high in flavanol antioxidants. Raw cacao has more antioxidant power than green tea and purple grapes. Choose high quality chocolate that is organic and make it a real treat after the meal.

If you have your eyes set on other sweet treats, try to get those made from natural sugars if possible and steer clear from the treats with synthetic chemicals. Avoid treats which are colored and flavored artificially. Just say no to those wild fruity flavors and crazy colored candies that just look too bright to be natural. Avoid the treats that say "diet" or "sugar-free", which are often sweetened with artificial chemicals. In general, if you are going to return to sweet treats, get in the habit of choosing treats which are made from wholesome ingredients which are better for you. Try those treats which that are labeled "organic" or made from a health-conscious bakery and only purchase what you can consume in one setting. I call these "healthy junk food." When you compare the organic whole grain, raw sugar cookie you'll definitely taste the difference when you compare it to the old Keebler™ version you used to like.

If the sugar craving is knocking at your door, and coming to get you after each and every meal, try some of these tricks. One of the best is to take a few raw almonds or other raw seeds and chew slowly to satisfy the sugar craving. Taking a small spoonful of organic peanut butter, almond butter or any nut butter and chew it slowly. Sometimes people do really well with a cup of hot herbal tea and add a little stevia or other natural sweetener. It can also be helpful to just brush your teeth with mint toothpaste and gargle afterwards. A piece of mint gum sweetened with xylitol can also curb a craving for sweets. Another trick is to taste something very bitter or sour. These two reflexes on the tongue stop it from wanting to eat anything sweet. A tablespoon of fresh lemon juice or a bitter herbal like "Swedish Bitters" tends to do the trick. All of these have proven to be helpful in kicking that addiction to sugar.

Snack Attacks and Big Macs

Some healthier snacks which are great for maintaining energy and low in sugar are a half sandwich or burrito, dried meats like beef jerky or beef pepperoni or smoked salmon which are NOT made with nitrites or MSG/autolyzed yeast extract or artificial flavors (ask your local health-oriented meat shop). Water-packed sardines on rye crisp crackers, a hard-boiled egg, a handful of raw nuts and seeds, an apple or whole grain cracker with some peanut butter or almond butter, or carrots, celery or any other veggie dipped in hummus or bean dip. You may even wish to eat half of your meal at meal time and the other half a couple hours later as a snack. As long as the food is not weighted heavily with carbohydrates or sugars, you can choose it for a snack option. (see list of snacks in the meal plan in the appendix)

You can still follow Nature's plan at restaurants as well. If you are going to a nicer sit-down restaurant, try to get your plate as close to the proportions of starches, protein, and vegetables as recommended earlier. Choose one starch only and keep it in a modest portion (that means if you choose to eat the bread, then no other starches at the meal). You may just say, "Scratch the baked potato and bring me a double portion of vegetables, please." If they can't do this, or you don't like their vegetable variety or preparation, order the entrée and order it with a LARGE side salad. Eat half the entrée and take the other half of it home for later. Actually, if you are with another health-minded person, this works out great if you both order your own green salad and then you split the entrée. You will be impressed with how satisfied you are, both with your meal and your bill.

If you are on the go, fast food is the last alternative. Not a good alternative, but it will do in cases of extreme necessity. It is preferable to choose a restaurant which offers food as low on the grease scale as possible, such as a sandwich which isn't fried or a burrito without cheese and sour cream. Whatever you choose, here is the trick: make sure you have with you a bag of celery, carrot sticks, or any other raw vegetable to eat with it. If you eat an equal weight of veggies with it, less fat will be absorbed and you will not have the negative effects you would if you ate it alone or with a side of fries. How about that for a tricky trick?

Remember to always resume drinking water an hour after you are finished with your restaurant meal. Restaurant food is loaded with sodium and other artificial chemicals including flavor enhancers; this is the major reason eating out can be so unhealthy for the body and so ADDICTIVE. You want to make sure you dilute these poisons with Nature's own solvent – water - so they can be excreted by your body and cause no undue harm.

What about those situations in which know you are going to imbibe but you have already "cheated" or exceeded your two free meals for that week? Well, this is where it gets tricky, but you can still slow the impact of these extra treats if you consciously combine them properly. Say you have a choice of a glass of red wine, a cup of chocolate mousse, or a piece of cherry cheesecake. Mmmm, sound good? In this case, watch the portion size of your treat so that it isn't the size of a dinner plate. Also… and here is the trick, choose a very large serving of vegetables at the meal to equal half the weight of the protein and carbohydrates. This time though, *in place of the carbohydrate starch, you should choose to eat your dessert treat.* So, in place of having a serving of potatoes, rice, or bread, substitute one of these for your dessert treat and eat or drink it after the meal. This will ensure that the sugars from the treat aren't absorbed too quickly as they are mixed with vegetables and protein. So, there is a way you can have your cake and eat it too!

Vegetables are an excellent source of fiber which, when eaten with food, mix with it to prevent large quantities of sugar or fat from being absorbed quickly. If you don't have access to vegetables, a similar effect can be made by drinking a fiber drink with the meal. I have formulated a fiber powder made with okra that is non-constipating and which can be used for weight loss or to bind up fatty rich foods which are not healthful. If taken before a meal, it will give a sensation of feeling full so you will eat less. If taken with foods which are not healthy for you, such as pizza or fried foods, it will bind the excess grease and pull it out of the body. This fiber also works great not only for those who want to lose weight but also for those with high blood sugars. Soluble fibers, when taken with food, bind with the excess glucose sugars and prevent them from being absorbed. The name is called Slippin Slidin™ and it is named for a good reason- to slip and slide that gunk right out of your body! (see Sources)

So that does it; treats are meant to be enjoyed, so go ahead and do just that - enjoy them once in a while. What you do the majority of the time is what will maintain your body's health. Remember, we are eating to live, not living to eat, although what would life be like without pizza or birthday cake once in a while? If it turns out that once in a while is getting to be more habitual and turning into several times or more a week, then you will want to make a plan or get a coach to make these cravings manageable.

With that, I will conclude these 21 days of Nature's Diet. It's been an honor and privilege to write this book and share with you what I have learned through my teacher Doc Ken, my patients, and by observing Nature directly. Continue onward with these healthy habits and you will continue to lock in your brain the patterns which will promote health for you and your family for the rest of your lives. - Be Well!

START NOW:

- "90/10 compromise": enjoy a meal of your choice or a treat of your choice a couple times a week.

- Pay attention to subtle hints your body is giving you when you return to the foods you have been avoiding. If you have a reaction, honor the body's wisdom and do not consume these foods any longer.

- Choose treats made from organic, natural ingredients as opposed to those with artificial flavors and colors.

- Snack on foods which are low in sugar.

- If you eat in a restaurant be sure to incorporate half the weight of the meal as vegetables and/or salad. This is particularly important if you are going to replace your starch with a dessert or if you have no choice other than fast food

Summary: This is what I'm doing up to this point, each day adds onto the next

Day 1: **Food awareness:** Keep a diary of my foods. I am accountable.

Day 2: **Water:** Sip half my body weight in ounces throughout the day.

Day 3: **Movement:** Some exercise performed every day. Note it in my diary.

Day 4: **Regular meals:** Eat about the same time each day.

Day 5: **Vegetables and Raw Living Foods:** 50% of total weight of your food.

Day 6: **Fruit:** Up to 2 servings of locally grown fruit daily (no fruit juice).

Day 7: **Carbohydrates:** One serving per meal combined with vegetables.

Day 8: **Protein:** One serving of healthy animal protein at every meal.

Day 9: **FAT:** Eliminate bad fats and add one serving of good fat per meal.

Day 10: Grocery shopping, food preparation, condiments, and serving sizes.

Day 11: Practical food combining: Mix, match, and rotate properly.

Day 12: Dinner or lunch type meals for breakfast (MENU IN THE BACK).

Day 13: Avoid Toxic Chemicals.

Day 14: **Supplements:** Choose whole food supplements to boost health.

Day 15: **SLEEP!** The same time each night and wake the same time daily.

Day 16: **BREATHE!** Filter your air and breathe deeply.

Day 17: **SUN!** Get some sunshine and optimize vitamin D levels.

Day 18: **Clean Naturally:** Remove chemicals hygiene & household products.

Day 19: **Cleansing and Detox:** Intestines, liver, kidneys, and fasting.

Day 20: **SEX!** Balance your hormones and communicate your concerns.

Day 21: **Enjoy a treat!** Two meals per week of whatever you want!

Appendix A
Meal Planner & Menu Ideas

Choose one protein, one starch, one fat and as many vegetables as you wish from the categories below. Use this to make your own meals. Menu ideas with complete meals follow this list on the next pages.

PROTEIN:
Choose one serving of animal protein
(about 3 ounces per meal)

MAMMALS	POULTRY	FISH
beef *free range or grass fed organic*	chicken	anchovy
buffalo	cornish hen	bass
elk	duck	caviar
goat	goose	cod
lamb	pheasant	grouper
moose	quail	halibut
organ meat *(liver, heart, etc)*	turkey	herring
rabbit	EGGS	mackerel
venison		perch
		rockfish
		roughy
		salmon
		sardines
		snapper
		trout

STARCHES:
Choose one serving of carbohydrate per meal

GRAINS *1 cup cooked*	ROOTS *Amounts listed*	SQUASH *1 ½ cups*	BEANS, PEAS *1 cup cooked*	PROCESSED GRAINS= *25-35 g/serving*
amaranth	beet *3c*	all winter squash	adzuki beans	corn tortilla *(3 small)*
barley	carrots *2c*	acorn squash	black beans	whole grain sprouted breads *(2 slices)*
brown rice	daikon radish *2c*	banana squash	black-eyed peas	tortilla chips *1 oz (20 chips)*
buckwheat	Jerusalem artichoke *1c*	butternut squash	fava beans	brown rice cakes *(4 small)*
corn kernels	parsnip *2c*	delicata squash	garbanzo beans	shredded wheat cereal *(3/4 cup)*
corn grits	potato *1c* *(any type)*	hubbard squash	green peas	whole grain pasta *(3/4 cup)*
kamut	rutabaga *2c*	pumpkin	great northern beans	whole grain corn bread *(1 piece)*
millet	sweet potato *1c*	spaghetti squash	kidney beans	rice pasta *(3/4 cup)*
oat meal	turnip *3c*	sweet meat squash	lentils	corn pasta *(3/4 cup)*
quinoa	yam *1c*		lima beans	rye crisp crackers *(8)*
red rice	yucca *1c*		mung beans	rice crackers *(1½ oz)*
rye			navy beans	sprouted grain bagel *(½)*
spelt			pinto beans	sprouted grain pita *(1 large)*
triticale			red beans	flax seed crackers *(1½ oz)*
wheat			soy beans	
wild rice			split peas	
			tofu	
			white beans	

EXTRAS:

apple sauce *1c*

rice milk/soy milk *8oz*
often contain 25-35
grams carbohydrate

coconut yogurt *6oz.*
soy yogurt *6oz*

VEGETABLES:
Choose one or more of the veggies below.
Remember the amount per meal should be equal to the weight of the protein and the starch.

artichoke	jicama
arugula	kale
asparagus	kelp
bamboo shoots	leek
beet *(raw)*	lettuce *(all varieties)*
beet greens	mushroom *(all varieties)*
bok choy	mustard greens
broccoli	okra
Brussels sprouts	onion
cucumber	parsley
cabbage	peas & pea pods *(raw)*
cactus nopales	peppers *(all varieties)*
carrot *(raw)*	radicchio
caulifower	radish
celery	rutabaga *(raw)*
cilantro	spinach
collard greens	sprouts *(all varieties)*
corn *(raw)*	squash summer
daikon*(raw)*	Swiss chard
eggplant	turnip *(raw)*
endive	tomato
fennel	turnip greens
garlic	water chestnut
ginger	watercress
green beans	zucchini

FATS:

Choose one serving of a healthy fat source below *(about 15 grams per meal)*
Oils= *15 grams per tablespoon*   Nut butters= *15 grams per 2 tablespoons*

extra virgin coconut	black currant seed
extra virgin olive	borage oil
raw nuts seeds/butters	evening primrose
almonds	fish oil
cashews	flax oil
chestnuts	hemp oil
coconuts	krill oil
filberts	palm oil
flax seeds	peanut oil
macadamia	sesame oil
pecans	walnut oil
peanuts	wheat germ oil
pine nuts	butter
pistachios	ghee
poppy seeds	tallow (beef)
pumpkin seeds	(raw dairy)
sesame seeds	
sunflower seeds	
walnuts	
olives	
avocado *3oz*	
coconut milk *2oz*	
fish serving *100g = 2500mg EPA = 8 capsules fish oil*	

FRUITS:
List of healthy fruit choices as an optional snack between meals:

Consider a serving to be approximately 1 cup of fresh fruit or ¼ cup for dried fruit

Apples	Grapes	Peaches
Apricots	Grapefruit	Persimmons
Bananas	Guava	Pineapple
Blackberries	Honeydew	Plums
Blueberries	Kiwis	Pomegranates
Boysenberries	Lemons	Prunes
Cantaloupe	Limes	Raisins
Cherries	Mangoes	Raspberries
Cranberries	Nectarines	Rhubarb
Dates	Oranges	Strawberries
Figs	Papaya	Tangerines
Gooseberries	Pears	Watermelon

MORE SNACK IDEAS:

Any meal can be cut in half and eaten 2 hours later in place of a snack.

- raw veggies: carrot sticks, celery sticks, raw broccoli, cauliflower, peppers, cucumber slices, turnips, rutabagas, jicama, etc.
  (raw veggies alone or dipped in: bean dip, guacamole, hummus dip, or nut/seed butter)

- one piece of fresh fruit (with raw nuts or nut butter)

- coconut milk yogurt, soy yogurt *(kefir for some folks)*

- beef jerky, pepperoni, smoked salmon
  (NOT made with MSG, or artificial flavors (ask your local meat shop)

- sardines (canned in water) on rye crisp crackers

- hardboiled egg *(not overcooked)*

- handful of raw nuts and seeds

- rice crackers with some peanut butter or almond butter

- apple sauce and raw yogurt/kefir or soy yogurt

- tortilla chips with bean, guacamole, hummus, or salsa dip

- olives *(tree ripened)*

- soup and flax seed or rye crisp crackers

- homemade fruit gelatin

- dried seaweed

- popcorn plain or with olive oil sprayed on

- half sandwich or burrito

CONDIMENTS:

- natural sea salt or mined minerals salt

- salt substitute (potassium chloride= No-Salt™ or Nu-Salt™)
  (for those with high blood pressure)

- tamari soy sauce

- herb seasonings: *(all herbs and spices may be used as condiments)*
  Mrs Dash, Spike
  powdered kelp
  Simply Organic dressing mixes

- unfiltered raw apple cider vinegar

- fresh lemon or lime juice

- all oils and nut butters listed above

- mayonnaise made from olive oil

- salsa, guacamole, hummus, bean dips

- organic mustard, organic ketchup *(read labels!)*

MENU IDEAS:

You may mix or match any of these ideas.
Remember there are no set breakfast, lunch, or dinner foods. Any meal can be eaten at any time of the day. Nature's Diet Cookbook will expand on this and have numerous meal plan ideas along with the recipe for each individual item.

3 oz baked halibut *1 ½ cups* winter squash with olive oil *2-3 cups* sautéed green beans	*2 medium* eggs poached *2 slices* Ezekiel toast with ghee *6 oz* fresh veggie juice *(50% greens + 50% carrot)*
3 oz roast chicken leg *1 cup* millet *1* steamed artichoke dipped in olive oil	*3 oz* broiled snapper *1 cup* sweet potato baked fries *2-3 cups* cabbage coleslaw
3 oz organic meat loaf *1 ½ cup* cooked peas/carrots with butter *2-3 cups* broccoli salad	*½ cup* whole grain oatmeal cooked with ½ banana, or *3* prunes or *10* raisins with *2 tablespoons* almond butter and egg nog drink on side: blend *2* eggs with almond milk
3 oz halibut *1 cup* brown rice cooked in coconut milk *2-3 cups* grated carrot salad	*2-3 cups* buffalo red bean chili *2-3 cups* cabbage-avocado-cilantro salad
2 soft boiled eggs *1 cup* black beans with salsa and avocado *2 cups* grilled onions and bell peppers	*3 oz* venison sausage *1* gluten free pancake with nut butter *6 oz* fresh veggie juice *(50% greens + 50% carrot)*
3 oz Cornish game hen *1 cup* medium potato with avocado *2-3 cups* Romaine salad	*3 oz* turkey breast *1* toasted sprouted wheat roll with olive oil *2-3 cups* lettuce, tomato, sprouts, cucumber

2-3 *cups* turkey bone broth soup with barley, veggies, and turkey 2-3 *cups* spring green salad with olives	3 *oz* lamb ribs 1 *small* baked potato with butter 2-3 *cups* Brussels spouts
3 *oz* organic beef liver 2 *small* corn biscuits with broth gravy 2-3 *cups* sautéed zucchini and onions	Egg salad on 2 slices sprouted toast (2 hard boiled eggs mixed with olive oil) 2-3 *cups* lettuce, tomato, sprouts, cucumber
3 *oz* venison steak 1 *cup* basmati rice 2-3 *cups* stir fry *(any veggies from list above)*	3 *oz* tilapia 1 *med* baked potato with tofu and olive oil 2-3 *cups* steamed veggies *(from list above)*
3 *oz* salmon lox ½ organic sprouted bagel with olive oil 6 *oz* tomato juice with greens supplement- *(Veggie Greens Powder drink- see Sources)*	3 *oz* Buffalo steak 1 *cup* yams or sweet potato 2-3 *cups* green beans
3 *oz* water canned herring 1 *oz* rice crackers and 1 *oz* hummus 2-3 *cups* raw celery and carrot sticks	3 *oz* wild cod fish 1 *cup* quinoa with avocado 2 *cups* steamed vegetables *(from list above)*
2-3 *cups* lamb and lentil soup 2-3 *cups* spring green salad with avocado	3 *oz* turkey breast 1 *cup* millet with olive oil and avocado 2-3 *cups* tomato and cucumber salad

3 oz roast beef and onions *1 ½ cups* roasted potato and carrots *2-3 cups* roasted zucchini-summer squash	*3 oz* lamb burger *1 cup* split pea soup *2-3 cups* carrot salad
2-3 cups beef and veggie soup *1 piece* corn bread and butter *2-3 cups* fennel and endive salad	*3 oz* chicken breast 3 corn tortillas *2-3 cups* grilled vegetables and avocado
3 oz roasted chicken breast *1 cup* white bean soup *2-3 cups* lightly roasted veggies	*2* low heat fried eggs *6 oz* coconut yogurt or soy yogurt *1 slice* whole grain toast *6 oz* fresh veggie juice *(50% greens + 50% carrot)*
3 oz broiled trout *2 cups* parsnip roots cooked *2-3 cups* European salad greens	*3 oz* duck leg *1 cup* basmati brown rice *2-3 cups* eggplant or portabella mushroom with tomato sauce
2-3 cups beef stew with potato/carrot/celery *2-3 cups* green salad	*3 oz* sea bass *1 cup* millet with olive oil *2-3 cups* leafy green salad with sprouts
3 oz organic turkey sausage *1 cup* whole grain cereal *6 oz* fresh veggie juice *(50% greens + 50% carrot)*	*3 oz* turkey breast stir fried *1 cup* rice noodles stir fried *2-3 cups* stir fried veggies- tamari seasoned
3 oz salmon pâté made with olive oil 3 tortillas with sliced tomatoes/ cucumber *2 cups* fresh garden green salad	*3 oz* deer, elk, moose liver *1 cup* lentils with onions *2-3 cups* stir fry *(any veggies from list above)*

Open face sandwich: *3 oz* mackerel or sardines pâté made with olive oil or olive mayo *2 slices* whole grain toast *2-3 cups* Tomato, sprouts, lettuce on side	2 poached eggs *¾ cup* shredded wheat cereal with rice, almond, soy milk *6 oz* water with green drink *(Veggie Greens Powder drink- see Sources)*
3 oz rabbit *1 cup* sweet potato with almond butter *2-3 cups* sautéed kale and collard greens	*3 oz* free range beef roast *1 cup* roasted yams *2-3 cups* broccoli-cauliflower steamed
3 oz wild rockfish sautéed in butter *2 ½ cups* rutabagas and turnips *2-3 cups* Arugula salad	*3 oz* free range beef ribs *1 cup* apple sauce *2-3 cups* sautéed kale and collard greens
3 oz sashimi *1 cup* rice noodles in miso broth *2-3 cups* seaweed salad	*3 oz* lamb *1 cup* pinto beans with tomato salsa *2-3 cups* asparagus
3 oz rabbit *½ cup* potato salad made with olive oil *½ cup* steamed beets with vinegar *2-3 cups* large green lettuce salad	HOMETOWN EGGNOG PROTEIN DRINK Blend *2* raw free range eggs *1 oz* soft tofu *(optional)* *1 tablespoon* flax seed meal *1 tablespoon* almond butter *½* ripe banana or *½ cup* frozen berries *(optional)* with oat, soy, rice, coconut, or almond milk

Appendix B
Sources

TRILIUM HEALTH CLINIC
Dr. Andrew Iverson, ND
5609 South Lawrence St
Tacoma, WA 98409
Contact us through
www.triliumhealth.com

Day 2:
Water filters:
*Removes physical contaminants and
electromagnetic contaminants with
multiple filtration levels and vortex to
make water that resembles Nature.*

For countertop and whole home:
AquaLiv™
PO BOX 1179
Rainier WA 98576
800.794.6976
www.aqualiv.net
*For a 5% discount to our readers off all
AquaLiv™ products- put in this code:*
trilium *at the time of ordering.*

For Shower Filters:
See our website
www.triliumhealth.com

Day 4:
Fasting and Detoxification Retreats

1) TrueNorth Health
Alan Goldhamer DC
1551 Pacific Avenue
Santa Rosa, CA 95404
707.586.5555
http://www.healthpromoting.com

2) Optimum Health Institute -
Austin Lou Ann King RN-
the very kind director
265 Cedar Lane
Cedar Creek, TX 78612
800.993.4325
http://www.optimumhealth.org

3) Optimum Health Institute -
San Diego
6970 Central Avenue
Lemon Grove, CA 91945
800.993.4325
http://www.optimumhealth.org

Day 7:
*Food allergy testing ELISA methodology
IgG, IgE and IgA testing available*

US BioTek Laboratories, Inc.
13500 Linden Ave North
Seattle, WA 98133 USA
877.318.8728
http://www.usbiotek.com

Day 9:
NATURE'S DIET COOKBOOK
www.triliumhealth.com

Day 10:
NATURE'S DIET COOKBOOK
www.triliumhealth.com

Dressing Mixes: Simply Organic
www.simplyorganicfoods.com

Day 11:
Food allergy testing ELISA
See Sources Day 7 on previous page

Day 14:
NATURE'S NUTRITION™ and
PHYTO-OX™ and VEGGIE GREENS™
For ordering information:
See our website
www.triliumhealth.com

Day 15:
goLITE® BLU Energy Light
Light Therapy
(check Costco)

Philips briteLITE 6 Energy Light
(check Costco)

Soleil Sun Alarm
www.soleilsunalarm.com

Day 16:
AIR filter:
See our website
www.triliumhealth.com

Day 17 :
Light Boxes:
See Day 15 on this page

Day 18 :
Water filters: for drinking:
See Sources Day 2

Economical shower filters:
See our website
www.triliumhealth.com

Day 19:
Fasting center : *See Sources Day 4*

Digestive Detox Cleanse™
Liver Cleanse
Urinary Cleanse
VEGGIE GREENS™
For ordering information:
See our website
www.triliumhealth.com

Book coming soon:
NATURE'S DIET
CLEANSE COMPANION

Day 20:
Prostate massagers:
High Island Health:
www.highisland.com

Salivary Testing (ASI)
Diagnos-Techs, Inc.
19110 66th Ave. S., Bldg. G
Kent, Washington 98032
Toll Free (800) 878-3787

Day 21
Food allergy testing-
See Sources Day 7 on previous page

Index

Symbols

A

B

C

calcium 30, 75, 82, 115, 132, 139, 172, 188, 190, 195, 204, 260

cancer 2, 19, 31, 55, 77, 92, 93, 98, 100, 108-112, 129-134, 139, 165, 166, 171, 183, 192, 198, 207, 222-224, 232-234, 241, 255-263, 265

candida 27, 63, 200
See also yeast

canned food 67, 68, 138, 139, 142, 161, 289

carbohydrate 51, 71-78, 141, 146, 149, 155, 208, 256, 278, 282
See also starch

cell phones 137, 138, 142

Chinese Medicine 7, 10, 54, 121, 194, 260

chiropractic manipulation 246

chlorine 30, 31, 32, 176, 182, 188, 231, 232, 234

chloroform 30, 232, 234

cholesterol 50-54, 57, 87, 92, 101-116, 130, 143, 160, 167-183, 234, 240, 252, 264

Cholesterol Oxidation Products (COPs) 107, 108, 130, 136, 143

chromium 193

circulation 26

cleansing and detoxification 243

cod liver oil 198

coffee 18, 27, 28, 46, 177-182, 208, 209, 212

cold pasteurization 136

cold-pressed oils 100

commitment letter 22, 25

constipation 241

cooked foods 54, 55

copper 188, 192, 204, 260

cortisol 106, 177, 253, 257, 264

cosmetics 182, 232, 233, 255

coumestans 256

craniosacral therapy 246

curcumin 201

D

dehydrating foods 64

denature protein 91

depression 10, 46, 165, 173, 207, 252

DHEA 106, 253, 263-267

DHT 253, 254, 266

diabetes 19, 51, 75, 100, 112, 114, 154, 160, 165, 174, 175, 183, 207, 222

diarrhea 54, 171, 183, 241, 271-274

diet diary 18, 22, 41

Di-indolylmethane or DIM 255

disinfection by-products (DBPs) 30

diverticulitis 171, 241

dopamine 161

dreams 5, 211

dry skin brushing 246

E

EGCG 65

Egg Beaters™ 109

Einstein 4, 8

electromagnetic memory
See resonance

electronic pasteurization 136

ELISA test 73, 274, 293-294

EMF Electromagnetic Frequencies 137, 138, 209

V

W

X

Y

Z